Your Relocation Solution

Your Relocation Solution

*Be healthy and happy
wherever you are*

Kylie Bevan

Health & Wellness Revolution

The opinions, ideas and suggestions within are intended for general instruction only.
The author is not offering medical advice or prescription.

Each person's physical, emotional and spiritual condition is unique. The contents of this book are not
intended to replace or interrupt the reader's relationship with a medical practitioner or other
professional. Please see your health practitioner for recommendations specific to you.

The author and publisher claim no responsibility to any person or entity
for any liability, loss or damage caused or alleged to be caused directly or indirectly
as a result of application or interpretation of this book.

ISBNs
978-0-9941830-0-2 MOBI
978-0-9941830-1-9 EPUB
978-0-9941830-2-6 PRINT

Editor: Natalie Montanaro
Typesetting: Steve Passiouras - bookow.com

For more information please visit healthwellnessrevolution.com
or kyliebevan.com

For information about quantity discounts, please use contact details as above.

To Rod, Emily and Talia
for embracing each new location
and for encouraging me to follow my dreams too

Foreword

I'm Robyn Law, also known as the Girl on Raw. I'm a formally trained raw food chef, coach, writer and speaker.

I've been an expat since 2005, living in the UK and Middle East. I currently live in Saudi Arabia, where I met my husband, also an expat from Australia. We're now raising our two children here.

This book would have been a godsend each time we moved.

Indeed, it is now, after almost 10 years away from 'home'. There are still plenty of challenges when living away from your comfort zone – some days it seems just too hard. Until I remind myself of the many things to be grateful for.

A process Kylie gently leads you through, like an angel showing you the most enjoyable route.

Within these pages Kylie reveals herself as the Expat Expert. She delivers your very own relocation solution, incorporating every element needed for a healthy life – food, water, exercise, relationships, purpose, spiritual practice and more.

I am a proponent of healthy living and that can mean so much to different folk. I am all about working out what works best for you and your own family - not just the food you put in your mouth but how you spend your days, and feeding your soul from within too.

I travelled professionally as a flight attendant for almost 9 years. I was always concerned with how I fuelled my body, and was always the first of the crew to find the local market after landing. Travelling for work or pleasure need not compromise health goals, and I wrote *Travelling in the Raw* to help others eat healthily when on a trip.

With the release of *Your Relocation Solution*, I contend relocating for work or pleasure is no different. Your health goals need not be compromised. You might even become healthier.

I am honored to introduce *Your Relocation Solution* to you.

Enjoy the read, take action and make the most of your healthy relocation!

Robyn Law 2014

robynjlaw.com

Contents

Prologue

Introduction

Being healthy and happy is a challenge for many of us, in our time-poor, highly stressed, demanding lives.

Eating healthily is only the tip of the iceberg.

Being healthy and happy is also about fulfilment in the other things that 'feed us'. Physical Activity. Career. Relationships. Creativity. Purpose. Joy. Spirituality.

Just contemplating fitting all of those into each week is a challenge.

Add events which are known life stressors[1], such as change of residence, change in work responsibilities, outstanding personal achievement, change in living conditions, revision of personal habits, change in schools, change in work conditions, change in social activities and change in number of family gatherings, and it's no wonder that relocating takes its toll on health and happiness.

This book aims to help this move, this exact relocation, be a positive one for you. The opportunity to start anew. Set good habits. Rediscover your passions. Embrace new beginnings.

The prime opportunity to truly look after yourself - as only you can!

About me

I'm writing this book while in Tonga. I'm here with my husband and two children. Visa requirements prevent my taking on health coaching clients in -country – a real downer for the few weeks, until I remembered that when one door closes, another opens.

I could embark on a new adventure of some kind.

Like write a book!

The perfect opportunity to combine my experiences with those of women around the world.

I've travelled a bit, aided by 15 years as a travel manager – visiting about 30 countries.

I've lived in 15 towns across Australia, as well as in England, Canada, Papua New Guinea and now Tonga.

I'm passionate about health, inspiring busy people around the world to tweak their lifestyles for the better, as owner of Health & Wellness Revolution, found online at healthwellnessrevolution.com.

I'm wife to someone who also likes to add value - not just be paid.

And I'm a role model for our two daughters - may their lives be healthy and happy.

Who is this book for?

This book is for women relocating and resettling anywhere outside their comfort zone, whether across town, across country, or across borders.

Without a doubt, male readers would benefit from reading this book too. It is written for female readers, however not exclusive to them.

Moving is challenging. Doing so in a healthy and happy way is even more so. This book will help smooth the bumps along the way.

What can you expect from this book?

Relocating can be isolating, with friends far away. This book is to remind you that you are not alone in feeling this way – and there are many things you can do to make resettling easier.

You'll be reminded of the importance of a support network. Of looking after yourself. Of noticing the silver linings, the lessons, the insights of living somewhere new and outside your comfort zone. Of the fabulously invigorating opportunity to start anew.

You'll meet women who have come through the experience with more gains than losses. They are the superwomen of this story.

And you, the heroine of your story, will get to know yourself better, too. Because nothing might change by reading this book – or everything might change. It's up to you to show up and do the work, knowing that what you need is already within you. With a little help from those whose experiences are showcased throughout this book, my role is to cheer you on.

Why me?

I've had two memorable turning points in my life—moments of realising there can be a different way.

The first was a diagnosis of Hashimoto's Thyroiditis, at age 40. Hashimoto's is an autoimmune condition, with 'members' increasing at an alarming rate. Way too big a topic for this book to cover, I've detailed recommended resources on the Health & Wellness Revolution website, healthwellnessrevolution.com.

This diagnosis set me on a new path, helping busy people take responsibility for their own health and happiness.

My second memorable turning point was finding almonds in Tonga - a country blessed with abundant fruits and vegetables, but limited options for packaged foods such as nuts, seeds and flour alternatives. With dietary limitations to support my autoimmune condition, finding nuts was pretty exciting stuff for this grain-free eater in a country with few alternatives to wheat and rice.

This was the moment I decided not only could *I* make a go of it in this new place, but that I could help others do so as well.

While the turning point for people relocating to a new place will vary significantly, I realised I could be the very person to help them recognise that moment – and to embark on a happier and healthier future, wherever they may live in the world.

Ways to use this book

With case studies, information and action plans, this book is designed to:

- ✓ be read in any order. Skip to the topic that you'd like to work on first.

- ✓ help you recognise many other women have felt like you – isolated in a new environment, unsure where best to find good food, let alone meet new friends. They made it through, and so will you.

- ✓ give you pause. To take time to examine how you are feeling, allow these emotions to be released. And determine how you'd *rather* be feeling. When you come across a question, it's probably not rhetoric. How would your honest self answer it? You might like to put these thoughts onto paper, in doing so clarifying what is at the heart of the matter. In words. Or doodle. Paint. Sing. Write a poem. Journal.

- ✓ be returned to. Promise yourself you'll do so, or diarise to ensure you remember, perhaps every three or six months. Reassess. Tweak. Enjoy.

- ✓ be a starting point. As tempting as it was to cover every possibility, and to provide in-depth information about every factor, I didn't want the length of the book to be daunting. ***Because this book may change your life.*** Read it in a day if you choose to. Allow it to be a 'leap pad' to learning more if you wish. Contact me if you need help, I'm happy to help further.

✓ connect you with others facing similar challenges and joys. Join the closed group Healthy Relocators on Facebook - just request to join group and your membership will be approved soon thereafter.

How to stay motivated

Ever started a project with gusto, only to have your enthusiasm falter?

May your health and happiness not be one of these.

This is how you are going to succeed.

One step at a time.

Peppered through this book are exercises to help you decide what you want and how to get there. To set goals – little ones and audacious ones - and outline the steps to get there. To figure out *why* you want that. To review. To be flexible – but dedicated to the big *why*. To celebrate successes. To surround yourself with positive people. To quiet that mean-spirited inner voice. To be proud of who you are. To practise self-care. To nurture friends who uplift you. To ask for help. To picture your perfect everyday day.

Tools like these will help you move from idea to action. One step at a time – in the right direction!

One moment more

Before we begin, please take a moment to think, what one thing could you do right now, to improve your health and happiness?

Do that.

Yep, right now. Before you read another page. I'm happy to wait. See you soon.

Top Ten Tips for Relocation Health

1. **Pick a word or phrase to focus on**. Mine is 'best choice available'. Whether it relates to food, exercise, home environment, career or relationships, this mantra gives me permission to make choices that relate to the *here and now*. Because that's where I am.

2. **Give yourself time to settle in.** In researching this book, women sometimes took months or years to enjoy their new location, often arriving via a satisfaction rollercoaster ride. Recognise every day as an opportunity to grow. Congratulate yourself for 'high' days and be gentle with yourself on the 'low' ones.

3. **Make the most of it.** Take a moment every night to recall or write down three things that you enjoyed today.

4. **Employ the help of a local** to show, or introduce you to, their favourite health practitioner, doctor, dentist, shopping places, hairdresser, restaurants, weekend location and areas to live. Ask lots of questions.

5. **Take care of you.** Get plenty of sleep. Treat yourself to a massage, facial or pedicure – DIY if the funds or service are not available. Meditate or write in a journal to help clarify your thoughts. Patiently remind your self-critic that you are out of your comfort zone and doing your best.

6. **Learn the local language.** This opens doors for cultural exchanges and new friendships, leading to greater respect, acceptance and opportunities. Learning a new language is also a powerful mind exercise, helping to alleviate stress and strengthen mental capability

7. **See the 'silver lining' in challenges.** Learn from any mistakes. How could you simplify what went wrong? Is there a way to solve that frustration? Who could support you in doing so? What else do you need – tools, advice, skills?

8. **Share your journey** with interested others, by way of a blog, social media, emails or phone calls. You may be amazed how many are in awe of what you've achieved. Recognise any negative feedback is their story, not yours.

9. **Spend time in nature**, with bare feet on park grass, walking along a beach, trekking through a forest or swimming in a lake. Time outdoors not only boosts feelings of wellbeing, by grounding and aligning, but also boosts vitamin D from the sun, vital for mental and physical health.

10. **Embrace the opportunity to become an even better you!** Why not take this new chapter of your life to purge poor habits and embrace new healthier ones.

Chapter 1 – Mindset

'Things work out best for those who make the best of how things work out.'

John Wooden

Shift your focus

Lukewarm shower. Rock-hard mattress. Blunt knife. Mouldy cutting board. 24hr crowing rooster. Aggressive dogs. Rats. Teary children. Refrozen meat other countries reject. Tiny fridge. Vegetables that wilt in a day. No dish-washer - or clothes dryer. A house so dirty we couldn't see out the windows. Reactions from each of us to pest control treatment at the house a few days before moving in, including vomiting and itchy eyes, throat and feet.

In contrast, children being called beautiful angels. Husband in fulfilling work. Time to complete unfinished projects. Baskets of fresh coconuts. The biggest smiles you've ever seen. And the most beautiful voices. Snorkelling in winter. Isolated beaches. Adventures. Fresh fish every day. Delightful traditional banquets. Mesmerising dancing.

What would you have chosen to focus your attention on?

As for me I alternated. There were certainly moments when my comfort zone, my home town, called - persistently.

But when I chose to be grateful for all we had, all that we didn't have wasn't quite so necessary.

I can recall the very day I decided to make a go of it. I also recall the day that I didn't think it possible.

On the good day, I stumbled across a new shipment at one of the many grocery stores that need to be visited to gather enough items for the week ahead in Nuku'alofa. I found a tub stacked with almonds, dried figs, gluten -free flour and dates. High excitement for a girl with dietary restrictions.

On the bad day, two eggs tumbled out of our fridge, and it rained on my washing. Yep, that was it. Even so, there were tears. The fridge was too small to stock enough vegetables, meat and eggs for four days of family eating. There was nowhere to put wet washing nor any hope of it drying before fading in intermittent rain and sun. I'd had enough of being stoic.

I was trying so hard to be everything. Mum, wife, cook, cleaner, shopper, connector, supporter, cajoler, health carer, safety officer, daughter, updater, business owner and blog writer.

Deep breaths. I made it through unscathed – exhausted admittedly, but oh so proud of success too.

If I could now give the 'me' who relocated to Tonga some advice before doing so, I would remind her not to make things more complicated than they need be.

For example, our experience in buying a car. Trying to save money by importing one, then not receiving duty-free as expected, having paid for a rental car for over two months while waiting for its arrival. Sure, we ended up with a better car by doing this, but also a fair bit of extra work clearing customs and the rest.

Also, by not allowing enough time to resettle, to find a house, sort out transport, connect utilities, restock the pantry and so on. Juggling clients, business and other projects added additional complication and therefore stress.

Next relocation I hope to recall the difference between optimism and unrealism – overstretching oneself is not healthy or happy.

Mindset tools

One way to put more focus on the good stuff rather than the challenging is to write three things you are happy for in a *gratitude journal*, just before bed. Going to sleep with positive thoughts not only promote a peaceful and rejuvenating night, but also helps you notice and attract more good things in your life. Some days it might be a push to come up with 'my morning cup of tea' or 'the rainbow that peered out after days of rain' or 'a roof over my head'. Other days it might be 'a truly connecting day with my family' or 'invited to share a celebration with a local family' or 'tasted a most amazing new food today'. Wayne Dyer, the 'father of motivation', teaches that whatever you are thinking about in the five minutes before sleep, before the subconscious mind takes over, is what will be dwelled upon until you wake[2]. Make sure your sleeping hours are spent on positive thoughts!

Another great mindset tool is known as *early morning pages*, a technique recommended by Julia Cameron for some twenty years[3]. In a nutshell, on waking, handwrite for three full pages or 20 minutes, whichever comes first, of everything that comes into your mind. Everything. No editing. No censuring. This is not for rereading by yourself or others, just a way to release those busy thoughts. Your words may be nothing of consequence, perhaps something like, *'I don't know why I am writing in this stupid journal, I'd rather have stayed in bed.'* Especially if it is that. Write it all down. Over subsequent weeks and months you'll probably learn more about what's really important to you than ever before. Many have been following this technique for decades, such are the benefits.

Of course journaling in general is a great way to let it all out, to become honest with yourself about the why's and how's. Don't hold anything back.

If you prefer a 'guided journal' to a blank page, I can recommend the *Integrative Nutrition Daily Journal*, available online from Amazon. With spaces for morning intentions and evening reflections, as well as weekly check-ins, monthly activities and guided exercises, it is a beautiful guide.

Another tool you might like to use is the *I am* statement. I am lovable. I am radiant. I am strong. I am funny. I am awesome. I am wealthy. I am worthy.

I am organised. I am present. Invite abundance into your life. Call what you really want into reality.

Alternatively, *I choose*. I choose to be powerful. I choose to be loved. I choose to be generous. I choose to be beautiful. I choose to eat healthily.

Similarly, affirmations are very powerful, even more so if said aloud and into the mirror. Even if you don't initially believe them! Louise Hay has written numerous books and resources about the subject[4].

Here are some of my favourite affirmations, from various sources:

> I truly, deeply, love and approve of myself.
>
> I am enough.
>
> I have many gifts to share with the world.
>
> I trust myself and my decisions.
>
> I am safe and all is well.
>
> I am happy to be me.
>
> I have what I need within me.
>
> I make the right decisions using my inner wisdom.
>
> I have the courage to step into my future with grace and ease.

Affirmations can help when feeling stuck, envious, worried, sleepless, lonely, angry or insignificant. Create statements that nourish you. Say them daily. You'll be amazed at the result.

Fiona's Experience

Kiwi Fiona has lived in the UK, the Netherlands, Australia and Italy, and most recently Tonga.

She loves meeting new people and embracing new workplaces. Fiona finds overseas stints interspersed with settled life satisfies her mild case of 'itchy feet syndrome'.

Chatting with Fiona, she needs to pause to think of her challenges in relocating. A little undesirable male attention and the associated chatter that travelling solo can attract, she suggests. The opportunity cost of the higher salary of staying put. Friends being spread over the world.

Fiona finds she 'rolls' with each location. The exercise varies, she incorporates it into everything she does. Here in Tonga she bikes everywhere rather than own a car, providing exercise and stress relief, while also costing much less.

She makes new friends easily, embracing the local social scene. She enjoys insights into other ways of life. Errands take up a small part of the weekend, then onto socialising, exercising and exploring.

Fiona's flexibility and mindset allow her to enjoy all opportunities that come her way – or if they are not apparent, to search them out.

For that she gives thanks to living in third-world countries, helping her keep a clearer perspective on life.

She asks 'Is that just a first world problem? And does it really help to feel unbalanced or stressed over it?' Most of the time, no.

The Rollercoaster

Just like anywhere, you're likely to have good days – and horrid days. But perhaps it won't be your local fairground type of rollercoaster when you relocate. More like the massive ups and downs of the *Colossos* in Germany, *Mean Streak* in USA or the *Tower of Terror* in Australia.

If you've not relocated before, you may be expecting an initial drop in satisfaction levels, then a steady rise.

My research suggests otherwise.

Lots of ups and downs before levelling out.

Knowing this makes it so much easier when one of those horrid days hit. You know you just have to ride it out. You know it will pass. And you're one day closer to all the pieces fitting together.

Your journey will be different, but it may be something like this:

1. **Preparing to leave.** You might feel busy, a little nervous, excited about possibilities.

2. **Arriving in the new location**. A little like a holiday, everything is new and different. You might feel motivated and energised.

3. **No longer a holiday.** Everyday tasks like grocery shopping and connecting utilities require so much effort and thought. You might feel de -energised and that you don't belong in this new culture.

4. **Uncertainty hits.** Was this really such a good idea? A dream – or a nightmare? Disenchantment and loss of confidence may follow.

5. **With a reality check comes the decision to give it your best shot.** It might be different but home – but that's exciting, right? This phase is one of trying out the local language and outings – and having a surprisingly good time. You may feel uncomfortable yet strong.

6. **Out of the blue something may bring you down,** perhaps happy or sad news from 'home' or a negative event. You may wallow in it for a day or two, but pick yourself right back up.

7. **Acceptance of your new place**. You are on the way to embracing the opportunities this relocation has to offer.

8. **There may be more slumps, but you meet them head-on now, knowing they are short-lived and you have the skills to surmount them.** You've got this relocation game down pat. You are tolerant of yourself and your new environment – in fact, you rather like what you've become here. OR perhaps this wasn't the best move for you, in your situation, and you go 'home', ready to appreciate all it has going for it.

Emotional health

Are you a glass half-full kind of lady? Or glass half-empty?

Sunshine with a few clouds? Or cloudy with a little sunshine?

Either way, sometimes you need a few strategies to get yourself out of a slump.

Now, when you're feeling flat, or depressed, or lonely, or frustrated, or anxious, knowing what to do to emerge from that feeling is not always obvious.

Which is not to say those feelings should be ignored.

But once you've recognised how you're feeling, accepted its validity, and considered what you could do to influence the situation, it's also nice to be able to move on to other moods – like delight, contentment and anticipation. Rather tempting, wouldn't you say?

So, why not grab a cuppa and write yourself a list of all the things that make you happy. Aim for 50.

Some suggested rules:

1. Your list does not need to be in order of importance. Let it all bubble out.

2. Include anything that comes to mind. Even activities that you do most days anyway. Some that take five minutes – a cuppa in the garden, or a warm shower, or a walk around the block. Others that can happen only occasionally. Perhaps several that haven't happened in a very long time.

3. Use colours, boxes, circles, images – make it yours.

4. Don't stop at 50 if your imaginative juices are working their magic.

5. Once finished, hang it up where you'll see it – inside your wardrobe door, bathroom cabinet or pantry door.

6. Use it every day, not just when you are feeling low. Prioritise joy in your life.

If you have children, they'll enjoy this activity too – our kids had a list of 60 each within ten minutes of my beginning mine! And it gives you something to point them toward when they say *"I'm soooo boooooored …."*.

Get into a routine

Some women enjoy routine more than others – but everyone needs elements of routine in their day. And the sooner you get into one in your new location, the better.

If part of your routine in your last location was a morning cuppa on the deck, you can make it happen here too. Or church every Sunday. Or wine and pizza night at the end of the working week.

Whether they are similar or different activities to what you did in your previous location, having regular, expected, enjoyable activities will help you settle in your new one too.

I have 12 habits and behaviours that I aim to achieve every weekday. This idea came from Leo Babauta of Zen Habits[5].

Ten minutes is my magic number, as once I begin, I often find time for more – thank you Leonie Dawson, creator of the Amazing Biz and Life Academy, for this tip[6].

1. Achieve my three most important tasks (MITs) first

2. Create before consuming

3. Be present and focused on each activity

4. Spend time on emails and social media just once per day

5. Exercise for 10 minutes

6. Clear and de-clutter home and office for 10 minutes

7. Say no to new projects and requests if sleep, exercise and play will be limited

8. Eat fresh fruit and vegetables

9. Meditate

10. Spend 10 minutes outside with bare feet

11. Feel and show gratitude

12. Smile

Could you benefit from a similar list of your own 12 *zen* habits?

Likewise, which habits can you let go of during this move? Which ones are no longer serving you?

You are the average of the five people you spend the most time with

Have you heard this expression before, that you are the average of those you spend most time with? Particularly in your social and home environment? It's really not surprising. Our emotions are contagious. Surround yourself with happy, positive, grateful people and you're more likely to feel that way too.

I'll elaborate on this and say you are also the average of how the ways you spend your time *make you feel*. So if you hate your job, read gossip magazines, or suffer comparison-itis when on social media sites, these negative emotions are going to spread across other aspects of your life.

So press the reset button. Or just press the stop button! Make an effort to introduce more positive stuff. Practise gratitude. Journal. Meditate. Laugh. Play. Especially outside. Surround yourself with people whose qualities you admire.

Allow your intuition to tell you what you need.

And crowd out the negative stuff.

Resilience

Resilience is your ability to cope with stress and adversity. It helps you bounce back from negative events.

Traits that build resilience are: strength in everyday and challenging times; sense of purpose or meaning; and experiencing deep enjoyment and genuine pleasure.

You can nurture these traits by changing the way you think. Notice how you are interpreting the world around you – and set it to positive if it's not already. Rewrite those deep beliefs about how things **should** be.

Is there a chance of rain – or mostly sunshine? Are your work colleagues frustratingly uncommitted – or are they balancing work and family commitments? Should shops be open on a Sunday – or is it refreshing to have a full day of rest and connection? Is a hurdle insurmountable – or can you muster all you need to overcome it?

Practise turning your thoughts from negative to positive every day – and soon it will be what comes naturally, along with resilience.

Andrea's Experience

Andrea has moved, on average, more than once every year of her life. Relocating more than 60 times across the UK, New Zealand and Australia, she's obviously gained some practice in choosing her ideal location, and now has a Sydney beach on her doorstep - literally.

Home for Andrea is fluid. It depends on who she is with, where she's at, where she's been, and where she feels she belongs.

In her most recent relocation to Australia, Andrea's satisfaction rollercoaster has been a wild one - from living with her partner's elderly parents for the first six months, to enjoying the great weather and exploring, to the uncertainty of choosing the right business, to finding a dream home, to establishing the dream business.

Missing friends and family across the world is challenging – but surmountable, especially as her business becomes more financially rewarding and location independent.

What Andrea has found most challenging is finding time for self -care. Not taking on too much. Always feeling there is too much to do to prioritise herself. Working crazy hours.

Having recognised her lapse in self-care, Andrea is determined to now also make time for herself. She already feels freer, more on purpose and more passionate about creating a business that supports her dream life while serving others.

Self-care is the final piece in the puzzle.

Self-care

Self-care can be elusive. Something you perhaps think you are doing, until you try to remember the last time you did something just for you.

Self-care can feel like a luxury you don't have time or money for. If that is the case, think of the *'air masks on an airplane'* rule - fit your own mask before that of anybody travelling with you. You can only serve others if you look after yourself.

Just in case this concept is totally new to you, here's a list to get you thinking.

- A warm bath with a book

- A body rub with essential oils

- A long walk along the beach or amongst the trees

- A massage, pedicure or facial

- A romantic or funny movie

- A trashy novel

- A fun and frivolous night out with the girls

- A peaceful meditation session in your favourite place.

- A trip to a place that renews and invigorates you.

Pick something that will fill your self-care tank. And make sure you do so regularly.

When it all gets too much

Not everything can be solved with desire and intention. If you are constantly feeling depressed, anxious or imbalanced, ask for support – from friends and/or medical practitioners. It may be that the reset button you need is medication. I've been there and many others told me afterwards they have been there too.

Life can be tough, and when your mental health is out of whack, it's can be too tough. If only medication will get you through, do that. Hit that part of your life on the noggin, because the next chapter is bound to be awesome.

Gains and losses

These are going to vary from person to person, and move to move.

Commonly, relocating women spoke of gaining cultural experiences, new places to explore and broader perspectives.

While losing proximity to long-term friends, having to re-learn where to go for what, knowing where they fit in, experiencing loneliness and feeling the lack of family support.

The best approach here is to appreciate the gains and address the deficits. What can be done to make the losses feel less enormous?

Emma's Experience

A Brit who has also lived in the US and Australia, plus a long period travelling in India, Emma has found moves within similar countries much easier than those with significant cultural differences - including the US where she found that a positive attitude can outweigh sincerity.

She is particularly aware of challenges in understanding the roles, expectations and opportunities for women in different cultures.

Emma's biggest challenge now is ageing parents so far away. With a requirement to remain in Australia after a marriage breakup with children involved, no longer can she choose where to live – nor can she accept a great job offer in France without applying for a change in a court ruling. Understandably, the thought of divorce and its ramifications never came into play when she and her now ex-husband relocated to Australia together.

In the meantime, Emma sees holidays as a luxury denied to many and gratefully welcomed, the opportunity to see the many ways in which we all live.

She sends a big thank you to 'new' friends. The ones who she didn't know when she moved seven years ago – who have cared for and supported her, and her children since then. She suggests when relocating to do everything possible to build relationships and seek like-minded people. Say yes to everything. Ask people about themselves. Look everyone in the eye. Find good friends. They are a source of joy and support in both the light and the dark times.

Emma is a big-picture girl. The lack of sustainability in our current lifestyle model is of much greater concern than what mass media spends its time on. For the same reason, she encourages her children to work out for themselves how to interact with others, manage life, give back, and stay true to their values - to do something worthwhile with this one precious life.

I love who I am. I love my life. Most of all I love my kids and my family. Shit is going to happen, frequently and unexpectedly, but that is ok, life is messy but it is a heap of fun. We really shouldn't worry too much about the small stuff because it is pointless. So my rules are simple.

Look after yourself.

Look after your family.

Do your best to look after the world.

Don't tell lies.

Be responsible.

Be kind.

Everything else is going to come and go. You can only make a decision at a certain time based on the choices you have available - and you will make the wrong decision sometimes despite your best intentions. Then you get to live with the consequences!

So I try to live by the above rules.

What can you learn from locals?

No matter where you live in the world, you can always learn something from locals.

As for me, in England I learnt the importance of getting outside, no matter what the weather or amount of daylight. In Canada I learnt how to drink a gallon of coffee each day - okay, admittedly not everything you learn will be beneficial. In Tonga, I learnt never to park a car under a coconut tree. In

Papua New Guinea I learnt to make my own call as to the safety of a nation - for the record, 99% beautiful people. In Bali, I learnt the importance of balance, in all their forms of three, such as right mind, right speech and right action.

The more you can integrate into local life, the more rounded your relocation experience is likely to be. Consider learning the language, attending social events important to the area and getting to know local traditions and customs.

Here in Tonga, and in many nations around the world, people often reply to a question with 'yes'. Often it is because they want to please, or it is the culturally polite response, whether true or not. It's not until you've become more accepted that you might receive a 'no' in reply. A friend has a recurring tip pop up on his phone each week – 'if you're hearing no, that's a good thing'.

Do you need a regular reminder of a cultural difference?

Travel tips when relocating

1. **Plan.** What restrictions are there for taking in food? How long do you expect before you find a farmer's market or fresh food store? What small appliances may make settling in easier, if you have other items coming later – perhaps a mini-blender, plate, cutlery, a can opener and sharp knife? Which snacks will help pass the time travelling, especially if you have children with you – perhaps fruit, dried fruit, nuts, muesli bars or vegie sticks? What supplies would be useful for you to have in order to avoid eating out three times a day when you first arrive? The blender, for example, could make smoothies, pasta sauces, dips, salad dressings, nut milk and juices. An insulated flask can keep drinks and soups warm or cold for the day. A water bottle may save you having to purchase bottled water.

2. **Drink lots of water.** This keeps you hydrated while also flushing out environmental toxins. It also helps remind you to move – at least to the bathroom.

3. **Check travel advice** and sign up for alerts with your consulate. Australians –smarttraveller.gov.au. New Zealanders –safetravel.govt.nz. US citizens –travel.state.gov. Other nations – Google travel advice for {residents of your country}.

4. **Purchase health or travel insurance.** Medical expenses can be astronomical for non-residents. As a travel manager I came across a couple who lost their home after one of them was hospitalised overseas.

5. **Check passport validity, visa requirements and recommended vaccinations.** And remember, even if you are not familiar with the local government laws, you are responsible to follow them. Ignorance is not an excuse, especially when it comes to getting out of jail.

6. Ensure scans or photocopies of important documents and additional contact details are left with someone not travelling with you, plus carry copies yourself.

7. **Research how to transfer money** if applicable. Fees vary widely, with bank fees often high. The following are not recommendations, simply suggestions - OzForex, World First, Currency Fair and KlickEx.

8. **During your first few days, walk a lot**. Studies show that walking aids positive mindset – and you'll see and take in so much more on foot.

9. **Research appropriate clothing** for your arrival, not just for the climate, but also for cultural respect.

Feeling at home

The sanctuary of your home environment can be very important, when all around you is new. If you are relocating with only some of your possessions, perhaps to furnished accommodation, consider packing items that will help you feel at home right away, safe and familiar. I brought bed covers, candles and books, and will next time add pictures, place mats, coffee mugs and towels. And maybe even curtains – but that's another story.

How can you put your stamp on your new place?

Anonymous Participant's Experience

Excerpts from my online questionnaire:

Where do you consider to be home?

Oh, not sure I feel like I have one.

Are you happy to be here {current location}?

Still unsure, I find lots of advantages but don't feel connected to the place.

What have been some of the joys for you personally?

To be really far from everything has provided me with some space, or zoom out perspective, to look at things from a different angle.

Setting goals

To determine how to get somewhere, you need to have an idea where you are going. Otherwise, you'll be like the Cheshire Cat in *Alice in Wonderland*.

> *"Alice: Would you tell me, please, which way I ought to go from here?*
>
> *The Cheshire Cat: That depends a good deal on where you want to get to.*
>
> *Alice: I don't much care where.*
>
> *The Cheshire Cat: Then it doesn't much matter which way you go."*

You don't need to call them goals if that word doesn't inspire you. They might be projects, plans, points of focus or resolutions.

And how you achieve them can be called action steps. Or actions, steps, processes, order, activities. Choose a word that lights you up.

A common technique for setting goals is to make them SMART – specific, measurable, achievable, relevant and timely.

You'll make them even more attainable by figuring out your why. I call this the Heart of the goal.

Why do you want to _____ (eat better / move more / find a job you like / make new friends / find time for spiritual practise / get along better with your spouse / improve health check results)?

Close your eyes. Visualise how you will look with this goal kicked? How will you feel? What will those feelings do for you? How will you know when you have it?

Picture yourself where you want to be.

An example might be: I will lose 5kg of bodyweight by December this year, *because* I want to have energy to play with the grandchildren, and I want to feel sexy and confident in a new red swimsuit.

Note the *I will* in the above example. Not *I'll try to*. Or *I should*.

I will do this.

There is space to set your goals in the action plan at the end of this chapter.

When you achieve a goal, reward yourself. Ensure it feels really good to have kicked that goal. Reinforce the desire to kick more. Your reward might be one of the self-care suggestions earlier in this chapter. Something that makes you feel awesome.

Remember, sometimes things get in the way of goals. Life happens. A key to goal success is doing the best you can, not focusing on the goal at the expense of everything else. For example, getting to bed late and neglecting sleep to carve out some me-time may not be the way to reach your end goal of feeling balanced and relaxed. Roll with the punches, be gentle with yourself, and use your intuition to know when you need to move the goal posts.

Lastly, the key to success with goals is to be accountable – enlist an account-ability buddy. A friend, a forum, a support group, a family member – or a coach.

Hence the Facebook group Healthy Relocators, free to join as a reader of this book. Just search Healthy Relocators, and request to join the group - your membership will be approved soon thereafter.

If you would prefer one-on-one or group program support, that's on offer too, see the options at healthwellnessrevolution.com.

One suggestion – only tell the 'right' people. Share with the ones who lift you up. Who will cheer you on. Who will help you get there.

Not the ones who might discourage and disparage. Only tell them when you're so committed that any negativity on their part only fuels your fire.

Because as Henry Ford said:

Whether you think you can, or think you can't, you're probably right.

Your Mindset Action Plan

This is where you'll commit to your own smart, heart goals.

You'll achieve them by being clear about what you want, why, the steps you'll take, and how you'll celebrate your success when you do.

In the **next 30 days** __/__/__

What	Why	How	Celebrate!

In the next **3 months** __/__/__

What	Why	How	Celebrate!

In the next **6 months** __/__/__

What	Why	How	Celebrate!

In the next **12 months** __/__/__

What	Why	How	Celebrate!

Chapter 2 - Relationships & Support Network

'See yourself in everyone.'

Wayne Dyer

You're in a new place. Suddenly you have two 'homes'. Perhaps more if you've moved before now, so how can you maintain contact with those you've left, connect with new friends, and also look after the people who have moved with you?

Let's look at these topics one by one.

Maintaining contact

Social media, internet and international phone networks have certainly 'shrunk' the world. The quality is often high, even in low-speed internet locations – it sometimes feels as though the other person could be right next door.

If possible, don't limit your contacts to email, social media and text. Pick up the phone and have a two-way, real conversation for a better connection.

Skype allows for 'free' calls if you have internet access, as do other VOIP (voice over internet protocol) providers. I've found Zoom to be particularly good, as well as free, with video, audio alone, group calls and the option to record. Also at the time of writing Skype has a $5 per month plan for 300 minutes of calls to mobile and landlines in 50 countries – this allows our children to regularly connect with their friends in Australia.

Skype also has Wi-Fi, currently with over 2 million hotspots worldwide. You just pay for the minutes you use, with your Skype credit.

My research uncovered frequent discontent with the quality of connections via email, phone or video calls. By that I mean the small talk, not the tiny delays between comments. You may find over time that lack of common experiences may make it harder to make conversation. Alternatively, it may give you interesting and varied viewpoints to cover. It all comes down to mindset, being open and authentic with the friends you would like to stay connected with, and being mindful of necessary frequency. Some friends you may be able to chat with once a year and it feels like only yesterday that you did so. Others you need to nurture by contacting them more often.

I know I need to 'warm up' with old friends, to regain those common threads, to feel my most real and familiar self. So, when I live overseas, I keep in contact often with group emails and social media posts. Having moved so very many times, there are friends in various cities around the world. Then I am gentle with myself and them when we cross paths again. I know that the friendship can be rekindled, but it may need time and intention to do so.

New friends

How good is it that you have the opportunity to meet some wonderful new people in your new place! Imagine the possibilities. It may take weeks or months to find these buddies, but once you do, you'll not be able to imagine life without them. Smile at everyone. Make eye contact. Ask them about themselves. Listen.

'Strangers are friends you haven't met yet.' What a beautiful concept. Some say I am too optimistic, but I truly do believe the best of everyone – and interestingly, I am not often let down.

Who do you already know who might know these future friends? Which groups could you join to find them – social, sporting, hobby, occupational or community?

Where do your sort of people hang out? The health food store? The swimming pool? The gym? The theatre? Do so too, you may find like-minded new friends.

Go where the positive people are - you are indeed the average of the five people you hang out with most. So don't hang around those who don't want to be where you are - it'll be a downward spiral that is hard to resist. Jump aboard the *opportunity train* instead. Hang around those who are embracing the cultural events, the social scene, the language and the local lifestyle.

That is, find friends by doing what **you** love to do.

- Invite new friends for coffee or lunch

- Gather people for a movie night or book club

- Join a group to learn the language, public speaking or a craft

- Take up a team sport

Natalie's Experience

Always longing to travel, then completing 40 months in the US Peace Corps in Romania and Tonga in her fifties, Natalie is passionate about cultural exchange. That passion brought her back to Tonga after a year in China teaching at a university.

The reasons for her relocation success?

She stays connected online, sharing what she's doing and seeing each day on social networks. As a CNN iReporter, she showcases the cultures and the people she meets with people in the US and all over the world[7].

She embraces customs, traditions and the local language so she can make friends beyond the expat community.

And she is generous to others, and they in turn are generous to her. For example, in Romania they so wanted her to stay they asked her what that would require. Thinking of her clothes frozen solid on the line in her mountain home, soon after the first clothes dryer in the village arrived as a birthday gift for her from the local mayor and church community.

But even with a positive mindset, relocating is rarely without challenges. For Natalie, this includes constantly giving away belongings, albeit happily, dealing with the packing nightmares and long flights across the oceans, and coping with long goodbyes which she never knows will be permanent or not.

"On top of all that an injury or illness to side track you is especially daunting."

Challenging, yes, but also gratifying beyond measure. Natalie is a Peace Corps advocate, a cultural exchange maven and a US citizen planning to live happily abroad for many years to come.

Relocating to your partner's home town

In the smaller world we live in, it is inevitable that many will connect with someone from another area or country.

Indeed, in my circle of friends, it's more common than not. It adds a wonderful variety to our combined experiences, skills, knowledge and insights.

While not stepping in the way of love and the ultimate connection, do pause to consider if long-term you are possibly, and then definitely, willing to compromise on living and working location. Consider all that this entails – education if you have children, distances from family and friends, language and new customs.

Ashley's Experience

Ashley met a local while a Peace Corp worker, courting for seven years in both his country and hers.

They've since married and had a baby – and are loving watching their daughter absorb the local language and culture.

Perhaps they'll return to the US in time – but for now the relaxed and slower pace of life, free from the bombardment of materialism and commercialism of the more developed world, is very appealing. Ashley can be a stay-at-home mum, as she was herself raised.

Yes, Ashley does feel the distance from family and friends, especially when missing an occasion such as a wedding or other important event, but so looks forward to the weekly Skype calls with her family.

Unfortunately, close female friends tend to come and go, given the transient nature of expatriates. Being asked for assistance with bills by extended family members is common, so for items such as school fees they allow the children to 'earn it' with a few chores.

Ashley nourishes herself mentally and physically with stroller walks with her daughter along the scenic waterfront and weekly yoga. She uses fresh and unprocessed local food, making almost everything herself. Overall, her physical health is just as good as when living in the US, with considerably less stress.

Ashley is keeping her toe in with her drafting and design career with freelancing projects, locally and overseas. She's also designing business cards, and designing and making greeting cards using local themes.

With clear communication, teamwork and acceptance of cultural differences, Ashley and her husband are able to bridge the cultural gap to maintain a successful mixed-nationality partnership.

Relationship dynamics

For some, relocating together may strengthen the relationship. For others, it may strain it.

I met my now-husband a month before he moved to Papua New Guinea. He was due to have already been there, however there had been a work visa delay.

After an exorbitant phone bill, $5 per minute at that time, we decided I should join him. I wasn't enjoying the job I'd just started, and we wanted to see if this brand-new relationship was going to blossom. For safety reasons I wore a wedding ring, and everyone assumed we had been together for some time - not just one month in Australia, then one month apart.

To be fair, Rod saw me at my worst in that first year. I wasn't very good at being a kept woman, and spent many evenings in tears - until I decided on a creative writing course by correspondence. My articles began being published in Australia and New Zealand, back in the days when the article and photos had to be posted to newspapers and magazines. I also started volunteering at a local school, playing squash with a girlfriend, playing competitive cribbage with Rod, and learning Pidgin.

When we announced we were returning to Australia to get married and start a family, our friends commented that if we could get through a year in a developing country together, we could get through anything. Perhaps so.

On the flip side, one of my research participants found the extra time together highlighted that they didn't enjoy each other's company so much anymore. Which may have happened over time in the previous location too.

An exercise I find invaluable for those wishing to better understand their close relationships, whether partner, child, parent or friend, is the quiz at www.5lovelanguages.com. Or purchase the book, by Gary Chapman. In a nutshell, we show our love in one or two main ways – with words of affirmation, acts of service, gifts, quality time or physical touch. We also like to receive it in one or two main ways. This quiz allows you to get to know yourself better, as well as those around you.

Relocating with children

This can be the toughest part for relocating parents. Because children are not *mini-me's*, nor can they necessarily see the long-term benefits of a move.

Rarely do children like change.

Many adults don't either.

Before you leave, involve children in the lead up to the big change – let them know why the family is moving. Let them help pack, decide what to take, and where to put their personal and precious things in the new location.

Perhaps try putting yourself in their shoes. Talk **with** them. If that's not easy to achieve, chatting while engaging in one-on-one activity may yield better results, like walking along a beach or playing a board game. Taking away the additional pressure of eye contact and body language may help their words flow easier. Or suggest they write it down to share with you. Or draw it. Adults often gain so much from journaling or freeing their creative side - children do, too.

Strengthen the family relationship. Perhaps start a family joke book. Or have a regular meeting so everyone is heard. Cook a meal together. Or allow each member the chance to pick an activity for the weekend.

Take mementos from the last location they can enjoy at the next, such as photos, certificates, farewell cards or a visual diary, so they can feel connected and purposeful. This is a fine way for children to have their own stories to tell, also priming them for a changeable future.

Help them keep in touch with old friends while encouraging opportunities with new ones. Arrange play dates and park outings with new people who also have children and this may just help you find new friends too.

Catherine's Experience

Not a stranger to relocating, having lived in the UK, Zimbabwe, Tonga and Australia, Catherine makes the most of a new location.

She volunteers or gains employment as the situation allows. She gets to know many, and becomes lifelong friends with a few. She exercises. She gets involved.

As a family, the posting eases the financial pressure of both adults having to work full-time to pay off the mortgage, as they would have to do if still in Australia.

Catherine's challenge this time around – settling-in the children. As friendly and energetic as they are, they didn't feel comfortable in school after many months. Stressed and concerned, Catherine decided to home school them. While this has been a challenge in itself, it was better than having unhappy children.

Catherine points the finger at herself, commenting she's not a natural mother. I contend. Like the rest of us, she's being the best mother she can be. And that is something to be proud of. Home schooling children? I'd say she deserves an awesome mum award.

Leaving children behind

Perhaps your children are older, schools which you or they would choose aren't available where you are relocating, or you're in a shared parenting arrangement.

So your children are staying behind.

How do you feel? How do they feel?

What can you put in place to feel closer in connection, if not in location?

Being left behind by a relocating partner

Perhaps your other half is being posted elsewhere, but you've chosen to stay for family stability, your current employment or study, or for health reasons.

Plan ways to stay connected. Talk about how everybody involved feels. Detail what to consider doing if an emergency or problem arises. Respect each person's role in this team arrangement. Ensure ways to share not just the good stuff but also the everyday and not-so-good stuff.

Be aware that there may be just as much readjustment when your partner goes, as when they return. Be gentle and understanding of each other's possible turmoil while this occurs.

Relocating solo

Moving on your own can provide its own challenges – and benefits. In researching this book I came across women who received unwanted or negative attention for doing so, which brought back memories of the same for me.

On the flip side, you need only agree with yourself as to how, when and where to go next.

Kavita's Experience

Australian-born Kavita has lived in the Maldives, Singapore, India, Hong Kong and Sri Lanka, more than 18 months in each. She is single and independent, having a wonderful time travelling the world, making new friends, living by the sea and keeping fit.

Meeting a man while relocating so frequently is on her mind. As is missing special occasions with friends and family 'at home'

– weddings, birthdays, new babies and other celebrations. For the first few relocations, Kavita found it hard to find her groove, putting on weight – she's now found routine and feels fit once again.

As she launches her own business, she's dreaming big, confident that she has been successful in what she has taken on before now, so will be again.

It's a step out of her comfort zone that perhaps travelling solo, and in doing so becoming independent, happy and aware of herself, has allowed her to take.

Get the support you need

Asking for help doesn't mean you're weak. It means you are wise.

Think back to the last time you asked someone for help. Chances are, they were delighted to give it. Because inherently we like to help. We like to give. It feels good.

It is crazy that it has become a badge of honour to try to do everything for ourselves. You **can** do anything – but not everything!

I'm not great at this myself – but I am working on it.

Care to join me?

Here's a list of the people and organisations you might ask for help. Some provide the service for free, others charge for the service. Search out those you can trust, personally and financially.

- Friends

- Family

- Social media groups and forums

- School community

- Church community

- Health coach

- Medical practitioner

- Relocation coach

- Relocation agent / consultant / specialists / service

- Helplines and Help Centres such as Lifeline and Beyond Blue

- And of course you can always Google it.

Your Relationships & Support Network Action Plan

Make a list of who you wish to stay in contact with.

- Daily?

- Weekly?

- Monthly?

- Yearly?

How will you stay in contact?

What can you do to meet potential new friends?

- Today?

- This week?

- This month?

What feelings are coming up for you here?

How will you help other people relocating with you find new friends?

Which support systems do you need to put in to place?

How will you begin?

Chapter 3 – Health Challenges

'You are as important to your health as it is to you.'

Terri Guillemets

Existing health conditions

Relocating with health concerns adds an extra dimension. Will you be able to find health practitioners you align with? Find the foods and supplements that support you? Live a lifestyle that nourishes you?

In my experience, there is so much you can do to ensure you gain more from the move than you lose, for three major reasons.

Firstly, if you already have people you know and trust on your health care team, there is a good chance they will be able to continue supporting you in your new location via phone or internet. Even practitioners you may only associate with hands-on, for example those offering complementary therapies such as reiki and kinesiology, often offer effective distance sessions and tests. In time you might learn of similar or alternate experts in your new location and add them to the mix.

Secondly, relocation is often an opportunity to keep the aspects of your lifestyle that you like, and ditch the rest. In my research, the number of people who adopted a healthier lifestyle after moving, far outweighed those who experienced a decline in health after their relocation.

Thirdly, you will benefit from the knowledge you gained in your last location and can add it to newfound information. Say you learnt how to make nutritious bone broth previously. You can continue to do that after relocating, and also learn how to prepare a local speciality that supports systemic health.

As for foods and supplements, eating local foodstuffs is best as they are freshest, picked for eating rather than travel, most environmentally friendly and in keeping with the season. For any extras, have you the option to use post, couriers or visitors?

Here in Tonga I've chosen to import chia seeds and quinoa to supplement what I can get locally, given my need to eat grain-free. However, the majority of my diet is what is locally available, as fish, coconuts, sweet potatoes, greens, bananas and papaya are abundant. I've been amazed how many different ways I can combine these foods!

I also import a probiotic powder, as gut health is vitally important, but also plan to make my own probiotic drink to solve that problem locally too. If ease of nutrition intake is the most important factor for you, I recommend the Miessence range of superfoods, one for each of probiotic, alkalising greens and antioxidants, as they also taste great – www.miessence.com/kyliebevan.

It would be remiss of me not to mention, it is possible to reprogram your genes[8]. Just because you have a health condition now, or your parents do, much of how you live affects how those genes are expressed. Improve how you are treating your body, your mind and your spirit to let your genes know their environment is on the mend.

My Experience

My husband and I took a break from overseas work to have children, mainly my decision, as I enjoyed the ease of first-world living with young kids. We always intended to introduce them to a developing country, to broaden their experience and educate them in making the most of what they've got – rather than always wanting more.

By the time we were ready to return to overseas work, I'd been diagnosed with an autoimmune, thyroid condition called Hashimoto's. Being the health nut that I am, I've chosen to address it with lifestyle change, in an attempt to delay medication, a life -long commitment once begun.

The suggestions for those with Hashimoto's would benefit most of the population. That doesn't make them easy or common. Remove the main inflammatory foods, beginning with gluten, then dairy, nuts and eggs if the condition doesn't improve. Increase anti-inflammatory foods such as fish, onions and garlic. Reduce stress. Increase opportunities for healing with more rest, a high -nutrient organic diet and frequent meditation. Take herbal supplements as recommended by a licensed practitioner. And have six-month interval follow-up tests to track hormone levels.

Some of these I can do more of in Tonga than in Australia, while others are challenging. The term gluten-free isn't known here, so there's limited eating out. Supplements are almost non-existent, so I've brought along supplies. Blood tests may not happen every six months, but this does allow me to justify an annual trip 'home' for them.

Really, when it all comes down to it, sending this autoimmune condition packing would take dedication no matter the location.

But there is absolutely no reason not to base my diet on the likely -organic, fresh, local fruits, vegetables and fish, available in abundance.

Every Sunday in Tonga is a mandated day of rest, and only the bakeries and churches are open. It's a day to relax, read, meditate, and spend time with family and friends.

I am living the life of my dreams - my weekdays are spent spreading the message of health and wellness, and weekends are for exploring with my family.

Now, if we could just tow Australia a little closer…

Health toolkit

Depending on your intended location, it may be worth taking some supplies with you:

- First aid kit with bandages, Band-Aids, sterile injection kit, antihistamines, pain relief tablets/gel and antibiotics.

- Homeopathy kit with guidebook. Trained practitioners would likely hit on the solution more quickly, however in my experience, self-diagnosis using homeopathic treatments has been incredibly successful, particularly for children. I use Ainsworths Essential Remedy Kit and other remedies from Homeopathy Plus, who ship worldwide - homeopathyplus.com.au.

- Regular medication and supplements with confirmation letters from medical practitioners for ease in clearing customs - check before you depart.

- Essential oils for anxiety, difficulty sleeping, immune support and more. I use Young Living - www.youngliving.com.

- Superfoods and probiotic powders for digestive support and nutrient intake. I use Miessence - www.miessence.com/kyliebevan

- A list of trained therapists where you are visiting.

- A list of websites for advice, such as travelmedicine.com.au and www.welltogo.com.au, and applications (apps) such as the Travel Health Guide.

Staying well while overseas

DO consider vaccinations before departure if travelling to a developing country.

DON'T delay getting medical advice for an illness just because you are unfamiliar with the location.

DO treat mosquito-borne and poor-food-and-water-borne diseases with respect by doing what you can to reduce the possibility.

DO take care with animals such as dogs and monkeys, as they may carry disease in developing countries.

DO take into account that sexually transmitted diseases are worldwide.

DO consider accidents and injuries while crossing roads, travelling in local transport, riding motorbikes and drinking alcohol – especially in countries that don't have strict driving-under-the-influence penalties in place.

DO boost immunity and recovery with natural diet and remedies. For example, the age-old remedies of garlic, citrus and horseradish for colds, flu and seasonal allergies.

Food intolerance

If you suspect a food intolerance and are not able to have diagnostic tests, you might like to consider eliminating then reintroducing the most likely candidates for clues and/or confirmation of what is causing the disagreement.

Food intolerance presents itself in many ways, via the skin, respiratory tract and gastrointestinal tract.

One of the best ways to check for a food intolerance is to eliminate it from the diet for 2-6 weeks, then reintroduce to see if symptoms return. Some people find that after allowing their body a break from a food group that had been causing problem, it can be consumed once again in moderation.

Food intolerance is a non-allergic food hypersensitivity. It can result from insufficient stomach acid or enzymes needed to digest the food, so your body is not able to absorb the nutrients from the food; or your body is not recognizing the substance as an actual food, therefore mounting an immune response.

The following most commonly cause intolerance:

- Dairy

- Gluten / wheat

- Salicylates, which are found naturally in many fruits (including strawberries, tomatoes), some vegetables (including capsicum, zucchini) spices, herbs, nuts, coffee, tea and wine.

- Soy

- Fructose

- Additives, preservatives, colourings and flavourings. For example, monosodium glutamate (MSG) is prevalent, especially in Asian countries and in restaurant meals, and can cause adverse reactions. Also common in processed foods is aspartame, an artificial sugar substitute.

- Citrus

- Eggs

- Seafood

- Nuts

- Alcohol

Many ready-to-eat foods are processed in factories which use nuts, soy, dairy and wheat, even if not in the item you are consuming. Check the label, but be wary and try to eat fresh rather than off-the-shelf.

Fran's Experience

Fran recently returned to Australia after two years in China.

The first six months were more challenging than fun, particularly the harsh climate and pollution, along with a vastly different language, governmental procedures and foreign customs. She worried about pollution exacerbating her daughter's asthma and felt guilty when her son didn't feel he was fitting in during the early weeks.

Then followed the adventure of it all – immersion into a city with a population larger than Australia, but contained within an area comparable to just one of Australia's capital cities. The buzz of street life, sense of community, the food, the bike-riding culture, and active older generations were a most enjoyable part of the big change.

Some challenges were ongoing. Missing family, especially elderly parents. Missing clean air, blue skies and nature at her doorstep. Lacking independence in not being able to drive there.

On days when things didn't go well, Fran coined them TIC (This Is China) days.

But also balancing those with what was on offer. Going out for interesting, great meals. Getting really fit with weekly yoga, tennis and riding her bike everywhere. Exploring greater China. Taking holidays overseas to sunny, nature-filled locations to get their nature fix. The growth of her children into global citizens, an amazing school community, and wonderful new friends. Finding that the pollution didn't exacerbate her daughter's asthma but that it actually improved, rarely needing her medication and shooting up centimetres.

Fran also had time to experiment with a gluten-free diet, hoping to solve constant stomach problems and bouts of gastrointestinal distress – with definite improvement.

While happy to be 'home', Fran and her family are so pleased to have had the opportunity to live in China for two years.

Your Health Challenges Action Plan

Are you currently doing all you can to support your current health?

How do you currently feel about managing and improving your health condition in this location?

What additional support, knowledge and resources do you need to help you do so?

What benefits for your health condition are on offer in this location?

What are the challenges with your health condition, no matter what the location?

What added challenges are there due to your new location?

What are you going to do about them?

Chapter 4 – Nutrition

'Let food be thy medicine and medicine be thy food.'

Hippocrates

Why do you eat?

Because you are hungry?

Because you like the taste and texture in your mouth?

To be social?

Because it is there?

It is interesting to note that when people eat, fuelling their body with the best possible energy source is not at the top of most decisions. Many people choose foods that are cheap, or easily available, or convenient, or tasty.

If you had an expensive sports car, you wouldn't dream of filling it with inferior fuel. You'd know that it would only operate at prime performance levels with the best fuel.

Your body is like that too. Nutrient-dense foods such as vegetables, fruits, quality fats and proteins will keep your body providing prime performance - balanced energy levels, immune support and overall health.

Fill it with processed foods, sugars and vegetable fats and your body will do its best to compensate. However in time your health, energy, vitality and body shape will eventually suffer.

How amazing is it that the body can be over fed, but undernourished? One reason for weight gain is the body constantly calling out for more nutrients - its owner might be filling their stomach and feeling full, but not feeding the cells what they need. The digestive system communicates to the brain that more nutrients are needed, which is then interpreted as more food required, rather than more **good** food required. Unless its owner is switched on, that may be more of the same, under-nourishing food. Weight problems, for some to the point of obesity, follow.

Or heart disease, Type 2 diabetes, hypertension or cancer.

So prolific is this way of eating that the term SAD has been coined – the Standard American diet. Or Australian. Or Anywhere.

Eating well in a new location

When you relocate, it can be even harder to eat well.

The food available may be very different to what you are used to.

Perhaps there is less available.

Or more.

Or it is hard to find, or expensive, or transport is difficult.

Or you are more time-poor.

Determining the best choices in a new environment is challenging.

In any case, my top tip is to talk about it. Ask locals what they love to eat in each season. Chat with market owners, butchers, restaurant staff and new friends. Google recipes - for example, 'breadfruit recipes', as I had to do for this readily available and tasty vegetable here in Tonga. Whatever the local produce, you'll be able to find a healthy way to use it.

Look out for a local recipe book, keeping in mind that traditional recipes may well be the healthiest option. It seems that no corner of the world has escaped the insidious sweep of processed ingredients such as white flour, white sugar and vegetable oils.

In times past, food was always seasonal and local. People didn't get sugar cravings because they enjoyed sweet fruit and vegetables when they were naturally available - not year-round. Hunted animals were eaten in their entirety and the choice pieces in many cultures were the fatty bits and organ meats - now proven to be excellent for good health. Food was also not always available, certainly not 24/7, so overeating was not as easy as it is now.

Is this relocation the opportunity you needed to rethink why you eat, how you eat and what you eat?

Kylie's Experience

Kiwi Kylie had 32 years in New Zealand before moving overseas to be with her husband. She left her podiatry career and six close siblings to join him in the family business in Tonga. She misses both her career and her siblings, but is thoroughly enjoying other aspects – particularly being in the same country as her husband, after five years apart.

Food availability has been a learning curve for Kylie on this small Pacific Island. Having been so used to popping down to the supermarket to pick up whatever her heart desired, or grabbing from the abundant sources of fast food, now she must go to five or more places to 'maybe' find what she's after. Kylie suggests that not having everything we want whenever we want it, feeling a little deprived and being forced to struggle a little, is good for us. I agree.

Kylie has lost 10kg since relocating a year ago, and looks fabulous. She puts it down to exercise and change of food. Here she cooks a lot more, and has someone to cook for, which has been amazing for her health. She's also recently started a vegie garden, another first.

Eating out

Even in the likely hectic first weeks, choose 'best available'. If you are eating out more than usual, look for the salads, vegetable dishes, and the least processed. If there is nothing on the menu that fits the bill, ask if they might prepare something for you. Always request sauces and dressings on the side. Ask for lemon, herbs and spices and if the restaurant doesn't have them, bring your own.

Availability and accessibility of fresh and dried food

Depending on how far you move from civilisation as you know, ingredients may be very different from what you are used to preparing. Be gentle with yourself as you transition. Expect mishaps. Eat out more often initially, if possible, and copy their ideas.

Our first 10 days here in Tonga were at a simple resort, and I was so looking forward to getting into a house and preparing grain-free meals. In my haste, I had to accept a large frozen hunk of tuna, as fresh fish was sold out. The supplied knife was blunt, so after hacking at it for some time, I had to put the whole thing in our only oven-safe dish – you guessed it, a tiny one. It looked hilarious, spilling over the sides. But instead of laughing along when my husband arrived home, peered in the oven and said 'What were you thinking?' I burst into tears. Thankfully it cooked just fine and made for tasty fish meals - many days' worth. However, it still quashed any cooking confidence I had in this new country with unknown greens, which irritate your tongue if not cooked properly; abundant fish, which had been expensive in Australia and therefore relatively rare for our family; over 40 types of starchy root vegetables; and coconuts. Four months later, I am loving what's available – but there have been some interesting meals during the learning curve.

If possible, ask locals before your relocation which foods might not be available, and if customs allow it, bring them with you. For example, into Tonga I brought, then had visitors bring, quinoa, chia seeds, dried berries and probiotic powders - these are not available locally, and courier delivery is expensive. Into many countries, however, online companies deliver for a reasonable cost, such as www.iHerb.com, which has a massive range of health foods and supplements. Do check restrictions with local customs so as not to lose it so close to being in your possession.

Petra's Experience

Petra was born in Tunisia to Dutch parents, and then moved to Holland for the rest of her childhood.

As an adult she has lived in the USA, France and Australia, before her current relocation to Qatar. Certainly some variety in that list! Benefits and challenges abounded in each.

Until Qatar, she quickly became part of the local community. This move was the first to feel like an expatriate. Even though she began with optimism, four months in, her satisfaction levels have plummeted, along with her health. For a lady who excels in making the most of new places, it's an understandably tough situation to be in. It's a completely new culture, she's catching new viruses, feeling less upbeat and less physically healthy, and finding it difficult to find nutritious foods in line with her own and her family's existing food intolerances.

The urge to return to the easy life of the previous location is strong. And not to be ignored. But also a decision not to be rushed into if possible (see chapter 12 – The Next Move). However, Petra has found a local farmer market. She's reading about healthy living, new foods, happiness and spirituality. She Googles nutrition information. She's taking time out for herself, taking a little puppy she found on the street to the beach in the early morning, and reading more novels. She's providing a warm, stress-free environment for her own family, rather than spreading herself too thin.

Petra is living within her environment, seeking out foods to nourish her family and herself. She's brought tools to help her do so, such as a Thermomix (a great food processor). And she's seeking knowledge so she can feel content, knowing that she's done everything she can to offer herself, husband and son, food and support to help them flourish in this new environment.

New kitchen / equipment

How easy do you find it cooking in someone else's kitchen, with different implements, pans and gear? If you find it challenging, as do many people, and you're able to, bring some of your own. Perhaps a food processor or blender, cake tin, baking dish, sharp knife, peeler, can opener and cutting board – that is, anything you regularly use when preparing food. This is even more the case if you might be renting a furnished house that may be stocked with everything the owners didn't want anymore. The day our shipped goods arrived was a massive boost to my enjoyment levels. Finally I didn't have to hack food with a blunt knife on a dodgy cutting board into a saucepan that burnt contents on contact with the stovetop.

Macronutrients

Fats are needed for the healthy operation of every cell of your body. For cooking, coconut oil, butter and ghee are best, given their high smoke point - other fats release free radicals on heating, which act as a wrecking ball for your cells. For cool to low heat uses, such as salad dressings and drizzling on cooked dishes, olive oil, macadamia oil and avocado oil are all good choices. Steer clear of vegetable oils such as canola, sunflower and rice bran - these require extensive processing and are very high in omega-6 fats. While essential to the body in the right proportion to omega-3 fatty acids, omega-6 fatty acids are over-consumed by most of us, which is strongly linked with many cancers and autoimmune diseases[9].

Proteins can be sourced from both animals and plants. Meat, eggs, fish, bee pollen, quinoa, chia seeds, nuts and leafy greens are all good sources. Grains, beans, dairy and soy can also be a good choice for those who can tolerate them. Choose organic, free-range, grass-fed and local when available and possible, as the health benefits of doing so are substantial.

Carbohydrates come from a wide range of sources - fruits, vegetables and whole grains through to sugar, flour and even alcohol. Complex carbohydrates, such as vegetables, are those that are digested over time by the body, slowly being released into the blood stream and converted to energy. Complex carbohydrates are desirable for long-lasting energy and satiety. Simple carbohydrates are those that cause a sugar spike, with insulin released in healthy individuals to counteract. Simple carbohydrates are not necessarily bad, for example honey and many fruits, however if eaten frequently, they are stressful for the body with 'sugar highs' and mood crashes.

Portion sizes

As a rule of thumb, pun intended, your own hand is a good guide for portion sizes for meals.

Remember for all food intake, quality over quantity.

Protein sources can be the size and thickness of your palm.

Carbohydrates can be the amount you could hold in two of your cupped hands if complex carbohydrates, and one cupped hand if simple carbohydrates.

For quality fats you may consume the equivalent mass of one or two of your fingers.

Acid / alkalising

All foods and drinks have an acidic or alkalising effect on the body. Studies suggest a ratio of 30% acidic to 70% alkalising foods to best balance the body's pH for health and longevity. However, the opposite ratio is more likely to be true for the average modern eater.

Vegetables and most fruits are alkalising for the body – this includes fruits such as lemons, despite their acidic taste, as once in the body, the effect is alkalising.

On the flip side, meat, dairy, grains, nuts, sugar, salt, alcohol and coffee are all acidic. When the body is overly acidic, it is stripped of minerals, and its owner experiences low energy, excess weight, acne, bowel irregularity and/or body aches. It becomes prone to weak bones, joints and muscles, kidney disease, heart conditions and diabetes.

Would you say 70% of each and every meal and snack you have is vegetables and fruit?

Congratulations if so.

A rocket up your bottom if not! This is one of the most important things you could rectify with your diet this very week. Michael Pollan, author of *The Omnivore's Dilemma* puts it this way - 'Eat food. Not too much. Mostly plants.' I couldn't agree more.

Bio individuality

One of key concepts I embraced from my health coaching course with Institute of Integrative Nutrition was bio individuality.

'One man's food is another man's poison.' We each need different foods to thrive, depending on gender, genetics, physical activity, age, health and environment.

Personally, the 'label' that matches my current way of eating is primal – but not strictly and not vehemently. That is, it works best for me right now, but that perhaps will change down the track. Primal/paleo to me means eating animal products, vegetables, fruits and occasional dairy, while eliminating or restricting grains and legumes. Give me a wheat item and I'm likely to have a migraine and/or fatigue tomorrow. A pretty clear sign that my body can't tolerate it right now.

But if I were to remove animal products from my diet, I'd have much less energy. As I would most certainly if I removed vegetables and fruit.

Dairy is more iffy – I'm a little like an emu with her head in the sand over dairy. Removing the gluten grains of wheat, barley and rye; and drastically reducing rice, oats and other grains, has been achievable. Also taking out dairy would be tough – but likely to be advantageous to my health, as it is another inflammatory, acidic food. For now, I've reduced it to the occasional bite of cheese.

How do I know which food items are causing me difficulty? By doing a 2-6 week food elimination diet. You can do the same. Experiment with eliminating a food such as wheat or dairy for 4 weeks and see if you feel better. If you've been diligent, if you choose to reintroduce a food after that time, you may experience physical or emotional symptoms such as digestive discomfort, fatigue, headaches, joint pain or anxiety. If not, but you continue to suspect possible food sensitivity, eliminate one or more of other common intolerances: grains/gluten, nuts, eggs, seafood, salicylates, yeast, alcohol, additives and fructose (as also discussed in Chapter 3). A health coach or dietician interested in healthy diet principles, can assist you on this journey.

Mary's Experience

Mary relocated with her husband to Australia after 25 years living in both Auckland and Queenstown, New Zealand.

It's been a good move for many reasons, including more satisfying, better paid work, in a bigger fishbowl.

Mary, like many other women who move, has experienced feelings of loneliness, insignificance and having to start again.

The first month was stressful with job seeking and numerous interviews, then the first year more exciting with a new job, friends and increased income. Now in her third year, Mary is feeling established, while still missing long-term friends and family. Making strong female friendships takes time.

Mary's physical and emotional health initially declined with the relocation, but now is the best ever. She's joined interest groups. She's sought and gained job promotions in line with her key interests. She's eating well, having overcome psychological eating – read more of her success at healthwellnessrevolution.com/testimonials.

Mary is moving forward in every aspect of her life – and looks and feels better than she has for a long time. She's an inspiration.

A one-week experiment

As a way of learning to listen to your body, consider eating a different breakfast, or lunch, every day for a week. Write down how you feel before eating, right after eating, and again two hours later. Note your energy level, your moods and your physical symptoms and consider if what you have eaten may have contributed to these feelings at all.

For example, breakfast options to compare might be eggs; meat with mushrooms, tomato or spinach (no bread); rolled oats; boxed breakfast cereal containing wheat; muffin and coffee; fresh fruits; fresh vegetables.

Lunch options might be a sandwich or burger; sushi or sashimi; lean meat with a salad or vegetables, but no grains or starchy vegetables such as potatoes; salad; muffin or scone; fresh fruit or freshly squeezed juice; wrap or focaccia; yoghurt.

You may discover sensitivity or intolerance to certain foods *at the moment*. Your body may need a break from these items to build up its tolerance again, to a certain point. This exercise gives you a better understanding on how important it is to connect what you eat with how your body reacts, physically and emotionally.

You can also do this if you are a smoker and wish to quit. Recognising the triggers that cause you to continue an unhealthy habit is the first step of the process.

Healthier alternatives

Commonly available	Healthier alternative for most
Margarine Canola, sunflower, rice bran oils	Butter, avocado or nut spread Coconut oil, butter or ghee if heating Olive, macadamia or olive oil for cold to warm use
Processed meats such as salami, bacon, lunch meats, hot dogs	Roast meats - organic and grass fed if possible Nitrate free bacon
Most breakfast cereals	Rolled or steel cut oats Mixes of nuts, seeds and dried fruit can be prepared once a week and stored in the fridge. Serve with yoghurt if not intolerant. Other breakfast options include smoothies, eggs, chops, vegie fritters, savoury muffins
White pasta	Quinoa Vegetable spirals such as zucchini, carrot, sweet potato

Bread / crackers / wraps	Lettuce leaves for wraps Spinach, mushrooms or tomatoes (with eggs) Salads instead of sandwiches Vegie sticks (carrots, cucumber, capsicum) with cheese or dips Wholegrain bread if not gluten intolerant
Wheat flour for baking	Coconut, almond flour or chickpea flour – proportions vary, begin with dedicated recipes such as at Elana's Pantry – www.elanaspantry.com
Ice cream with additives and 'numbers'	Blend frozen fruit – honestly, it's that easy. Try banana, mango or frozen berries. Most become creamy after 3 or 4 minutes in blender. Add egg white if needed.
Packet snacks such as chips, biscuits	Fruit – add variety with different fruits or method of preparation - fruit salads, cooked fruit, dried fruit, fruit skewers, frozen berries …. Nuts – almonds, macadamias, brazil, cashew Homemade popcorn
Breakfast and muesli bars	Check the ingredients panel, some are better than others. If you don't recognise all the ingredients, try making your own - easy, economical and you know everything that goes in!
White sugar	Raw honey, stevia (without fillers), dates, real maple syrup or raw sugar if you must
White table salt	Himalayan or Celtic salt

White potatoes	Sweet potatoes, pumpkin, squash
Milk	Rice milk, nut milk – available from supermarkets, homemade is even better
Cheese	Nut cheese such as cashew
Soft drink, cordial or alcohol	Coconut water, freshly squeezed juice, water kefir, kombucha, herbal tea, water

Not sure where to begin? Why not swap one line each week?

- Google some recipes, such as 'wheat free muffins'.

- Do your grocery shop with this in mind.

- Once the items are gone from your fridge and pantry it will be easier to resist.

- Take your healthier alternatives to friend's places to ensure you can stay true.

- Have a healthy snack in your bag in case you are out longer than you expect – I have a handful of almonds in my handbag all the time.

Other than food, what else feeds the body?

Relationships, spirituality, movement and play each receive their own chapter.

No less important are these:

Sun

Many people around the world are deficient in Vitamin D, which the body produces when exposed to the sun.

Our large houses, shady decks, long work days and busy lives keep us indoors more than ever before – and when we do venture outside, we're 'sun smart' in summer, we obediently 'slip, slop, slap' as a health promotion in Australia termed it – we slip on a shirt, slop on some sunscreen, slap on a hat.

Then in winter, we expose less of our skin to a weaker sun.

Nor can our diet provide enough. The best sources are fatty fish, mushrooms and eggs, providing only a small amount of vitamin D3.

One study estimates 73% of Australians are deficient in vitamin D, the active part of which is a hormone, and essential for healthy bone formation, muscle strength and our immune system.

To find out if you are deficient, ask your general practitioner (GP) for a blood test. Ideally, you'll be at the upper end of the normal range, but with so many people who are deficient, the *normal* range is low.

Boost your levels by:

- Soaking up those beneficial rays of sunlight. Aim for at least three times per week, 10-20 minutes at a time – or when your skin turns the lightest shade of pink. The darker your skin, the longer you'll need. Use sunscreen if planning to be in the sun for longer than that.

- Drink one tablespoon of cod liver oil a day.

- Take a good quality probiotic such as Miessence FastTract (gluten free) or InLiven, - for more information visit www.miessence.com/kyliebevan.

- Take a good quality Vitamin D3 supplement daily.

Sleep

Not many adults get the recommended 7-8 hours for healing and recovery. One sign that you are not getting enough is requiring an alarm clock to wake at sunrise, refreshed and ready for the day. Another indicator is low melatonin levels in saliva testing.

Poor sleep results in fatigue, irritability, poor concentration, poor memory, stiffness and lowered immunity. Relationships suffer, bad habits are acquired, your physical performance is hampered and you are more likely to put on weight!

The old adage 'an hour before midnight is worth two after' is regaining ground, after being swiped to the side in favour of our modern busy lives. This is particularly valid for many women who enjoy the quiet productiveness of evenings, then struggle out of bed in the morning, a sign of adrenal fatigue.

To get a great night's sleep:

- Reset circadian rhythms by doing only calm, technology-free, artificial -light-free activities after sunset. And on sunrise, get out into the daylight, a signal to your body chemistry to give you a hand waking up.

- Aid your body clock by keeping to the same bed times – sleeping and waking - each day, including weekends.

- Feel physically tired, having exercised during the day.

- Reduce or eliminate all light, Wi-Fi and noise disturbances from your bedroom. Use curtains or wear an eye mask; leave your phone and tablet in another room; use ear plugs; use a battery-operated clock.

- Avoid coffee, tea, chocolate, 'energy' drinks and large meals in evening, and for some, all afternoon.

- Keep your bedroom cool, about 18-20°C or 65-70°F, by opening a window or using a fan if a warm location.

- Take a warm bath or shower before bed, so your body temperature can drop, cueing sleep. Adding magnesium flakes to the bath, or spraying magnesium oil on your skin afterwards, is also relaxing and rejuvenating.

- Drop a little lavender or ylang ylang essential oil on your pillowcase.

- Drink a cup of camomile tea before bed, as long as a bathroom visit isn't then required during the night.

- If you wake during the night, try deep breathing or meditation to relax you back to sleep.

- And if it is your children who are having trouble falling asleep, try guided meditation from smilingmind.com.au/

Dr Rubin Naiman says sleep is the easy path to enlightenment - "sleep is serenity, sleep is inner peace"[10]. He suggests many of us are not only sleep-deprived, but also dream-deprived, risking depression, suppression of creativity and/or living mired lives. Dreaming allows us to live in a bigger, richer world. He suggests thinking about dreaming to encourage more of it. Wake up slowly, linger for 4-5 minutes in that semi-conscious state, mull over remembered dreams, and record them by writing or talking about them

Interestingly, in my own research, many commented they were benefitting from more sleep after their relocation. Sounds like a good opportunity to reset healthy habits to me!

Creativity

Creativity is something many of us let go of, when the pressures of being an adult swamp us – things like getting a good job, paying the rent / mortgage, sharing our time between self, partner, friends and family, renovating, and so on.

Think back to when you were a kid. What was it that you could lose all sense of time when doing? Would you like to pick it back up again now?

Or think of something you've always wanted to give a go. Learn a musical instrument. Learn to draw, to paint or to sing.

Albert Einstein said 'Creativity is intelligence having fun'.

And like relationships, purpose and movement, creativity is key to feeling balanced and satisfied in all aspects of your life.

Allow your creativity to shine, through artwork, music, cooking, building, creating, writing or whatever your heart desires. Enjoy being unique. Have some fun!

Your Nutrition Action Plan

Which foods will you eat more of?

Which foods could you eat less of?

What is one thing you can do right away to improve your nutrition intake?

Is there anything stopping you from doing so?

What can you do to solve that?

What else 'that feeds you' is not getting enough of your attention and time?

Think relationships, spirituality, movement, play, sun, sleep and creativity.

What can you do to improve whatever is lacking this week?

Chapter 5 - Movement

'If you want something you've never had, you must be willing to do something you've never done.'

Thomas Jefferson

Incorporating physical activity

I've suggested you read this book in the order that suits you.

Confession: Because I've written this book in the order that suited me.

This chapter was one of the last ones.

Why? Not because it's a difficult topic to talk about.

Instead, because it would have been hypocritical to write before now. I've only just started following my own advice, four months into our time in Tonga. And thinking back to other relocations, I did the same in each.

It's funny that physical activity is the thing I find hardest to incorporate into my life when we move. It gives me energy. It makes me feel good, with the release of endorphins, serotonin and dopamine. It means my clothes continue to feel good. And it has loads of other health benefits that I'll detail further below.

But because I do enjoy it, it's easy to slip into the trap of getting all the less pleasant things done first. I find I can get to the end of my week and realise

I've perhaps fitted in one walk or one yoga session. Of course, this is not nearly enough.

I've been checking out the options and have absolutely no excuse not to jump back into regular physical activity. Here in Tonga, that will be a run/walk with Hash House Harriers – a worldwide social group 'with a running problem' - once a week; yoga once a week (twice if another class is introduced); a foreshore walk with a friend once a week; and resistance training with weights at home twice a week. Plus incidental exercise time when market shopping, playing with the kids and any community events.

Yay!

Adding movement to your weekly routine

If you find it hard to exercise, my top tip for incorporating physical activity is adding it into your everyday. You know the score – park further away from work or school, take the stairs not the lift, ride or walk to nearby errands rather than taking the car, clean the house with energy and speed, get into the garden to weed and dig, and/or set your computer to remind you to get up and move once an hour.

Here are 26 more ways to move. Why not set yourself the challenge to tick off a new one every week for the next six months?

1. Stand on tiptoes when waiting in a queue.

2. Hold plank position during TV commercials, where you hold a straight position with only elbows or hands, and feet or knees, on the floor.

3. Dance around the kitchen between fridge, bench and oven while preparing dinner.

4. Surprise your kids, partner or friends by putting some music on and inviting them to dance.

5. Do push-ups until the kettle boils for your daily cup of tea or coffee.

6. Spice up your walk with a few short sprints.

7. Fly a kite.

8. Chase your dogs or kids around the yard.

9. Do pelvic floor exercises while waiting at the traffic lights.

10. Do 20 star jumps on the hour every hour.

11. Do 10 squats before your shower each day.

12. Have more intimacy if in a relationship.

13. Write a to z with each foot while seated.

14. Drink more water while at your desk, to ensure more trips to the bathroom.

15. Plan a walk date rather than a coffee and cake date.

16. Play target Frisbee, solo or with others.

17. Offer to take a neighbour's dog for a walk.

18. Use a hand fan rather than electric.

19. Skip using a rope for 5 minutes.

20. Dance around the lounge room a-la Tom Cruise in *Risky Business*.

21. Run in the water, at pool or beach – laugh at all passer-by comments.

22. Bounce on a trampoline.

23. Wash and polish your car by hand.

24. Make an enormous sandcastle with any child who wants to join you.

25. Find a park with exercise stations.

26. Do yoga sun salutations on rising.

Gabby's Experience

Gabby has lived in Papua New Guinea (PNG) and Tonga for the last nine years.

PNG was extremely challenging for the first year. Arriving in Port Moresby with a 2-year-old and 3-week-old, having left a cosy life in Australia, with supportive parents around the corner and sisters in nearby suburbs.

The main challenges in PNG were malaria, adjusting to the climate, safety and security and ultimately loneliness. It put a huge strain on her married life, as well as the stress of adjusting to a new baby in the family.

Gabby says the joy of their two young children kept their focus on what could work for them, rather than what wasn't working for them - children being great reminders of what is important, and what is not.

Moving to Kokopo, on an outer island of Papua New Guinea, was a further challenge - more isolated, and with a third baby.

Gabby found a sense of belonging when she became involved with the children's school. This was their first exposure to school, and she wanted it to be positive. The school needed help, and she could see potential.

She also recognised the need for something for herself, beyond teaching at the school. Missing the group exercise classes available in Port Moresby and Adelaide, and being a health and physical education teacher, with the encouragement of a few friends, she began teaching yoga.

This further entrenched her sense of belonging to the community. Gabby became known as ' the yoga teacher', which gave her a laugh, as she was herself still learning. She found women were very grateful for a little taste of home every time they came to her class.

Gabby has continued teaching school and yoga classes in Tonga, which gives her a sense of purpose and enjoyment. She loves the kids she teaches, along with the amazing teachers she works alongside. It broadens her outlook on life.

She's also found that planting a small garden in each new place helped her settle in, even when she didn't feel she wanted to. She suggests all relocators try that, even if it's just favourite herbs in a pot.

By keeping active, by feeling fit, healthy and strong, Gabby has been able to overcome the challenges, while embracing more opportunities.

Best choice available

As with food, it's a good mantra to follow. Best choice available.

What can I do to move more in my new location?

- Moving can be very energetic and exhausting - packing boxes, lifting suitcases, cleaning the old and/or new accommodation – you'll know when physical activity is needed again.

- Ask new friends how they stay active

- Call health units for a list of recommendations

- Keep open to new ideas. Shugyo, a form of Tae Kwon Do, was certainly not on the list of possibilities for our children before they arrived in Tonga – but within weeks they were facing their first grading test.

Be social

Exercise is a great way to bond with new friends, whether a team sport or individual. A common interest always helps conversation flow.

Barbara's Experience

New Zealand, England, France, Tunisia, Italy, Greece and Tonga have all been home to Barbara, some for a few seasons, others for many years.

As a chief executive, Barbara is in Tonga to help support export growth of agricultural products.

Like many expats, including myself, establishing an exercise routine, eating healthily and avoiding too much alcohol amidst a wealth of social activities ranks high on her list of challenges. Also, Barbara is here without her partner, who works in New Zealand, so is missing their lifestyle together as well as their mutual friends.

Barbara's satisfaction levels are climbing as she reaches the three -month mark and she actively addresses the challenges. She's enjoying the demands and variety of this new project. She's enjoying the cultural experiences. She's committed to eating healthily and drinking less alcohol.

And she's arranging an international swim event, from the main island to a nearby one. A very good way to get fit – and to be social.

Why exercise is important

- Improves body appearance, increasing confidence and self-love

- Boosts energy and vitality, enhancing enjoyment and prolonging life

- Lowers stress hormone levels, reducing risk of depression and anxiety

- Helps balance blood sugar levels, reducing risk of diabetes and weight gain

- Strengthens respiratory function, reducing effects of asthma and respiratory illness

- Helps elimination of toxins through bowels and skin, protecting against some cancers

- Strengthens immune system, reducing illness

- Raises good cholesterol, lowers blood pressure and reduces arterial inflammation, while reducing the risk of heart attacks and strokes[11].

What type of workout?

For maximum fitness in minimal time, Mark Sisson, author of Primal Blueprint, recommends regular, brief, intense strength-training sessions and occasional all-out sprints for optimal gene expression and broad athletic competency. Many others agree. So there you go, no need for hours on the treadmill any longer. In fact, that's just inviting boredom and repetitive strain injuries.

Mark Sisson offers a fitness blueprint, free, for subscribers to his site – plus lots of other awesome resources and well-researched articles[12].

I can also totally recommend the workouts of the day (WOD) that Kim Morrison posts on Instagram a few times per week. This is an example, please Google the moves if they are not familiar to you:

- 10 burpees

- 20 push ups

- 30 crunches

- 40 mountain climbers

- 30 second plank

- 20 tricep dips

- 10 slow squats, holding 3 seconds each

In a nutshell, keep variety in your exercise and incorporate more movement into every day. Do a mix of long low-impact activity (such as walking or cycling) for endurance and emotional health; bodyweight exercises (such as squats, lunges, push ups and pull ups) for strength and fat-burning; and fast/intense workouts (such as running or swimming sprints) for agility and speed.

Your Movement Action Plan

What form of physical activity are you going to do this week?

Are you incorporating one form of resistance (weights or bodyweight exercises), one form of endurance (long walk or run) and one form of interval training (fast then recovery in pool, on bike, on foot)?

Does it involve a schedule change or increased funds?

If so, how will you manage this change?

What support do you need to make it happen?

If necessary, think outside the square – swapping services if financially strapped, such as scuba lessons for child tutoring; or time if hours are of the essence, such as walking meetings.

Chapter 6 - Purpose

'The meaning of life is to find your gift, the purpose of life is to give it away'.

Pablo Picasso

Skye C's Experience

Australian-born Skye first ventured beyond home shores on her honeymoon – and was disappointed to discover that Phuket was not all that different to Australia.

So she later welcomed the opportunity to relocate to Tonga. Two years in, and she's not sure if she would describe Tonga or Australia as home, as she feels she belongs in both.

Not that it's been easy. Relocating and resettling with husband and five children. Not being permitted to drive the project car, Skye's weekday transport is by foot. Not being able to carry much food means making the most of hubbie's choices from a limited supply, such as thick-skinned chicken and fatty beef. And not having reliable internet made for interrupted study days and difficult connection with friends and family elsewhere. Not having a working oven, well-flushing toilets and hot water at times has also been challenging.

But Skye admires the local habit of being happy – handling dramas and rising above them. This attitude encouraged her to rethink her own everyday incidents, which naturally come with location changes.

So why does it now feel so satisfying for Skye? Firstly, not being permitted to work has allowed for university study and painting. Secondly, living in-country has opened doors to volunteer her current learning in the field of psychology through Red Cross. And thirdly, she's meeting like-minded people who are realising their own creative dreams.

For Skye, the relocation gave her the opportunity to recognise herself as a mum – and as *Skye*.

Now Skye and family hope to stay in Tonga long-term – she and her husband have found their purpose, their calling, their own individual and family gifts to the world.

As Skye says, *'it was important for me to be more than an accessory to my husband's role here'*.

Clarity of role

In researching this book I came across a lot of women who were 'expat wives'. Trailing spouses. Accompanying partners.

Handbags. Stylish, but of little consequence.

Wow, what a concept! We allow our partner freedom to make a difference, accept fulfilling work or take on a new challenge – and belittle ourselves for doing so.

As if we are a passive accessory to the move.

I'd like to refute that viewpoint.

Because marriage is a team effort. If one person is bringing in an income, the other is likely to be managing the home, or caring for children, or providing support in a multitude of other ways.

He or she is not an accessory, however beautifully they may adorn the other's presence.

Those very spouses may have left a career in the previous location and be restricted from working in the new. Or may be needed for other functions in the team effort, as it is in Tonga where shopping for necessities can be a day in itself. Or they may see a higher calling in voluntary work in the new location.

In any case, none of the above terms sit well with me. I'm happy to announce that my husband and I chose to relocate as a team. Neither of us requires me to accept accessory status in that arrangement. Indeed in the next location it may be reversed – but we'll still be the same team.

Difference in paid role or workplace

Many people relocate for a more interesting or better paying job. Excellent if that's you too.

I have a mantra. Yes, another one.

> If you don't like something, change it.
> If you can't change it, change the way you think about it.

Margaret Engelbreit

If you are enjoying your role or the benefits it brings, great work.

If you're not, take some time to think about whether it is time for a change. We'll return to that idea shortly.

Alternatively, think of ways to enjoy what you are doing more. What frustrates you? Can it be changed? What would make it better? Who or what might be able to help you do that? Is it a cultural difference that perhaps you'll get used to in time? Might there perhaps be a silver lining to your frustration?

As one example, perhaps the work ethic where you've relocated may be considerably more relaxed than you've experienced in the past. In this scenario perhaps attention to detail and level of output is frustratingly low for you. What will you gain from feeling stressed and bothered by that? Very little, I'd suggest. What will you lose from adding in extra hours yourself to even it out? A lot, I'd suggest. Would it be possible to do the best job you can, leading by example, instinctively knowing that busting a boiler would not have encouraged change in others? This moderate version may not either, however at least you've not lost your own health and happiness in the process.

Think of what might tweak your role for the better. Is it shouting your workmates to afternoon tea? Bringing in a pot plant and your own pretty coffee mug? Suggesting to a colleague a walk and casual chat during some lunchbreaks? Is it in embracing a realistic workweek?

And remember, you've changed roles once, you can always do it again.

Choosing to leave may also be the 'best choice available'. There is no shame in recognising that you need to move again to move forward.

Margaret's Experience

Margaret is employed as a volunteer by an international organisation, so earns local pay. No stranger to life in a developing country, her most recent relocation has been challenging. A job that wasn't as expected, dirty homestay accommodation, staff not coming to work and meetings being cancelled after time spent preparing.

Gains such as fitness from riding a bike for transport and cultural appreciation haven't been able to outweigh the losses, including financial.

Six months in, she rates her satisfaction level at 3 out of 10, disappointed that she hadn't achieved more.

So Margaret has decided to move on.

To write a book about some of the inspiring women she's met.

Margaret is embracing a new opportunity.

Opportunity to start afresh? Or consolidate, study, research, write?

Let's look at defining your passion and purpose. Is this relocation the opportunity to do something new? The thing you are great at? And that you love doing? And that others value? This is your sweet spot. Find this, and you'll never 'work' another day of your life.

Honestly. Probably sounds bizarre. But it can be done. I am, and many others are. We've found that beautiful place where everything aligns and we are offering to the world not only what we are best at, but that also fills us with pleasure.

The exercise in the following action plan will help you clarify what this might be.

Making a difference

Once upon a time, there was a wise man who used to go to the ocean to do his writing. He had a habit of walking on the beach before he began his work.

One day, as he was walking along the shore, he looked down the beach and saw a human figure moving like a dancer. He smiled to himself at the thought of someone who would dance to the day, and so, he walked faster to catch up. As he got closer, he noticed that the figure was that of a young man, and that what he was doing was not dancing at all. The young man was reaching down to the shore, picking up small objects, and throwing them into the ocean. He came closer still and called out "Good morning! May I ask what it is that you are doing?"

The young man paused, looked up, and replied "Throwing starfish into the ocean." "I must ask, then, why are you throwing starfish into the ocean?" asked the somewhat startled wise man. To this, the young man replied, "The sun is up and the tide is going out. If I don't throw them in, they'll die." Upon hearing this, the wise man commented, "But, young man, do you not realize that there are miles and miles of beach and there are starfish all along every mile? You can't possibly make a difference!"

At this, the young man bent down, picked up yet another starfish, and threw it into the ocean. As it met the water, he said, "It made a difference for that one".

Loren Eiseley

Sally's Experience

Sally's story is one of contribution as an adult to the community that shaped her childhood, Tonga.

As a primary-school age child of expatriates, Sally's childhood was similar to what it may have been in New Zealand – swimming lessons, Brownies, chocolates from Grandma in the mail and local schooling.

There were of course memorable differences, such as learning Tongan dance and wearing traditional costumes for a performance, riding in the back of trucks and horseback riding with rice sacks for saddles and ropes for reins.

And horrifyingly, one time hiding behind the couch when burgled by a man with a machete because the security guard had fallen asleep, and another time holding her breath when a drunk man came into her bedroom.

In the main, however, she, her sister and their friends learnt how to make their own fun in an idyllic environment.

Now a legal advisor in her 30s, Sally felt the call to return, to contribute, to help make Tonga safer. She sees Tonga as having so much potential, with kind people sharing what little they have, opening their homes, making everyone feel welcome. She's learnt to appreciate what others take for granted - drinkable running water, safe places to cross the road, laws against violence in the home. She loves the order, the traditions and the influence of the churches on Sunday.

Sally says Tonga has come a long way in 30 years, with roundabouts, paved roads, rubbish bins, cafes, elections and development – *'something I came to be part of'*.

In the workplace as a paid volunteer with a non-government organisation, she's enjoying helping in small ways that are greatly appreciated, being innovative and being listened to. In her spare time she's also helping children who are terrified of the sea learn to swim, as well as volunteering at a local school.

So strong was the call to return that she has left her daughter in the care of her sister while she takes on this role, bringing her over for school holidays. Contract requirements, safety concerns and being a single parent made this a necessity, and it is working out for all involved. Her daughter is loving having four 'siblings', her sister more involvement with her niece, and Sally is following her dream.

An example of thinking outside that square box.

Your Purpose Action Plan

Draw three large circles, interconnecting at the centre.

In one, write everything you are good at, not restricting yourself to work-related items. Perhaps cooking, travelling or reading. Aim for 20 or more.

In another, write everything you like doing. Your passion. The things you lose all time doing. Again, 20 or more.

In the third, write everything the world values that you can do. 20 or more.

In the centre, consider anything that appears in all three. On another sheet of paper, write all the ways you could offer this gift to the world, all the varieties of work that these encompass.

Which one is your purpose right now?

How could your current career align? Or, how could you create a new career path?

What do you stand for?

How do **you** want to be remembered?

How do you want **your work** to be remembered?

Chapter 7 – Play

'The body heals with play, the mind heals with laughter,
and the spirit heals with joy.'

Proverb

When did you last laugh? Muck around just for the sake of it? Reclaim your inner child? Throw off your serious hat?

Since when does being an adult mean having and being no fun?

What are you going to do about it?

Can you pull it off without excessive alcohol intake?

You are not alone if not. Society teaches us to be adult = to be sensible.

Unfortunately sensibility can be a little dull. Here are some ways to reclaim your inner child.

- Play chase with a (friendly) dog.

- Invite girlfriends over for a musical movie – think film *Mamma Mia!*

- Hire a comedy movie.

- Play a board game such as Pictionary.

- Play charades.

- Borrow some kids for some backyard games, such as pass the orange, balloon bulls eye, follow the leader, and so on.

- See an animated movie.

- Paint like a famous artist is in you.

- Or finger paint.

- Sing whatever you like.

- Turn the music up loud and dance in your living room.

- Break out the karaoke machine.

- Jump on a roller coaster.

- Learn to surf, or do Zumba, or hula hoop.

Nicole's Experience

Nicole has tasted city and country life in Queensland and the Northern Territory of Australia, with a move every few years of her adult life. It's now hard to know where to call home.

In some places she has been happy, others not. Being close to the beach was lovely - but expensive. One country town had great people, housing and a reasonable cost of living – but husband wasn't happy. Other towns had little to do, were sometimes hard to make friends, and there was little choice when you didn't like your job.

Overall, Nicole says relocating has broadened her horizons, has provided great job opportunities and she's learnt about other cultures. Gains 1 losses 0.

How has she coped so well? By doing whatever was on offer in each location. In Thargomindah, socialising, playing sports and participating in community events. In Darwin, eating out, visiting markets, and visiting national parks. At Mt. Isa, volunteering at the music shack and surfing the net. In Cairns, hiking, camping, visiting attractions and group exercise on the esplanade. In Charleville, playing lots of board games.

Nicole always remembers how to nurture herself with play.

Your Play Action Plan

Just do.

Chapter 8 – Spirituality

'Where your attention goes, energy flows.'

Various

What is spirituality?

Very few terms have such differing definitions as this one.

May I suggest connection with something greater, through religion or nature?

Meaningful activity or transformation?

What does it mean to you?

Does it involve meditation or prayer or mindfulness or study of religious texts?

How would you like to be and feel as a result of your spiritual practice?

More loving? Compassionate? Tolerant? Self-aware? Insightful? Strong?

Do you find the time to practise the forms of spirituality that feel right to you, that feed your soul? Do those around you understand its importance for you? Is it something you're not sure how to develop?

Perhaps this is another reason for your relocation, to discover differing practices, be open to new concepts, come across new beliefs, strengthen or challenge your own.

As with every segment of your new life, be gentle on yourself and those around you, and open to opportunity. Without even knowing it, spirituality may have been a void that you've been filling with less satisfying substances. Perhaps what you've been looking for is here, in your new location.

Brenda's Experience

Born in South Africa and relocating to Tasmania, Australia, as an adult, Brenda's major challenge has been discovering how and where she fits in, adapting her approach to fit an almost "old school" culture.

She found this particularly necessary with business marketing, where she wished to build trust and credibility as an industry expert.

Of particular note is how Brenda's emotional health has improved since relocating. She feels much more positive, grateful and spiritually connected. She's stronger, more authentic and compassionate.

She still has moments of vulnerability, so far from the support of old friends and family, and she wouldn't say she's happy all the time. Her eating habits and exercise have slumped.

But she likes to focus on the gains. Safety. Freedom. New Friends. The opportunity to find her purpose – and to fulfil her dreams.

Brenda admires anybody who has struggled and pushed through. I hope that includes herself!

Brenda is now helping others fulfil their dreams, coaching them in creating a thriving business with purpose.

What does Brenda feel is carrying her through the challenges, to come out in a better place?

Her beliefs. She has a strong faith – and knows how to use it.

Silence

Whatever your form of spirituality, you are likely to benefit from silence. This is when we allow our God, our intuition, our inner calling, our inner self be heard.

If you are new to listening for this voice, you may like to begin by training your mind with guided meditations. While not silent, this may help you learn this new skill.

I began with free recordings from the Chopra Center for Wellbeing. There are quite a number of free offerings on the net, to help you discover what form works best for you.

Meditation is shown to reduce anxiety and stress, enhance immunity and give you a stronger connection with what is within you – a form of self-discipline not always used to its advantage. Unheard but speaking volumes.

Reena's Experience

Reena has lived in small town Australia, capital city Australia, Canada and India.

She now lives in a scenic area of Australia, surrounded by nature, national parks, wildlife, bushwalks and friendly cafes. A 'tree change' relocation.

Plus, with her 'soul home' being India, Reena travels back and forth with her business.

Readjusting has taken time. Constantly trying to see everyone resulted in exhaustion. Business arrangements also created stress until the partnership dissolved. Health conditions flared.

Reena is now embracing the stillness and bliss of her location. Her spiritual side.

The walks in nature. The silence. The peace. Yoga. Meditation.

And is feeling all the better for it.

Your Spirituality Action Plan

This simple tool has revolutionised some lives already. Introducing the well-being planner.

It can be used as a planner, for the week ahead, or a tracker, for the week that has been. This can also be downloaded from healthwellnessrevolution.com, under free resources. Enjoy!

NOURISH YOUR BODY	Mon	Tue	Wed	Thu	Fri	Sat	Sun
Breakfast							
Lunch							
Dinner							
Snacks							
Drinks							

NOURISH YOUR MIND	Mon	Tue	Wed	Thu	Fri	Sat	Sun
Learn							
Appreciate (gratitude list, favourite part of day)							
Relax (bath, massage, sleep)							

NOURISH YOUR SPIRIT	Mon	Tue	Wed	Thu	Fri	Sat	Sun
Connect with self (meditation, breathing, journal)							
Connect with greater (religion, garden, nature)							

NOURISH YOUR WELLBEING	Mon	Tue	Wed	Thu	Fri	Sat	Sun
Move							
Play							
Relate (call, write, in person)							
Achieve Important Task 1 Important Task 2 Important Task 3							

What are you having trouble making time for?

Why might that be?

Chapter 9 - Finances

'It's never about your resources, it's about your resourcefulness.'

Tony Robbins

Relocation costs

Moving to a new location is often expensive. Even if within the same state, there's the removal van, new utility connections, obligatory deposits and rental security payments or house deposit. Move interstate, and there are driver's licenses, car registrations, insurances and more to change over. Move overseas, and add air fares, shipping costs, customs charges, vehicle purchases, temporary and permanent accommodations, school fees, phone/internet plans, currency exchange and more.

Whether or not you have the opportunity to negotiate inclusions as part of the employment offer, these are some of the items to consider:

- Accommodation costs, in a safe and convenient part of town

- Temporary accommodation for arrival, plus meals out

- Rental bond, lease cancellation fee - or selling and buying property cost

- Relocation costs of items to take with you – possibly including car, boat, bikes, pets

- Storage cost of items to remain in 'home' location – plus insurance

- Healthcare cover

- Initial transport and trips home

- Education fees

- Rental management costs if you own property at 'home'

- Living costs such as groceries, eating out, energy, internet, laundry and fuel

- Location pay / hardship allowance / security allowance

- Risk of currency fluctuations

- Currency transfer fees

- Partner's ability to work – availability, visa requirements and cost

- Health club memberships

- Foreign language tuition

- Tax and financial advice

- Absentee voting

- Local social security obligations

Budget

If you're moving to a new country, the cost of living can be fairly tricky to determine. Sure there are plenty of comparative reports for most cities around the world, and they will give you ideas. However, availability and cost of accommodations can skew the budget considerably, so factor in a large portion of your budget for housing. If you then find something more reasonable, there'll be less pressure than the other way around.

Save

Is there going to be potential to save in this new location? If so, is this a good opportunity to pay additional from the mortgage, or boost your superfund, or put some aside for a rainy day? Or will spare money be used to explore your new location? Knowing and committing to what you want this relocation to achieve, especially if you are travelling with a partner, is worthwhile. You want to gain more in some way, either in your bank account or your memory bank.

In my research, I met women across the financial spectrum, from earning a fraction of their 'home' salary, to many times more. Some were 'getting ahead' financially, others were dipping into their savings, and others were having a grand old time spending a whopping big pay packet. Just like in any city of the world.

How would you like your financial situation to look six months after this relocation? One year? Two years? Do you need to make any changes to what you earn, and what you spend, to get there?

Liya's Experience

Oman, Germany, Singapore and Australia have been home to Liya – 11 moves all told.

What she loves about where she is now? Full citizenship rights. Being able to live independently. Nature. Friendliness. A wonderful school community. The prospect of knowing a country well enough to read between the lines. The joy of building a life.

But what a journey to get to this point! Having to start over and over again. Finding friends. Feeling culturally tone-deaf. Being the sole parent for long stretches of time while her husband worked overseas. Many times feeling very alone and lonely. Transitioning back into the workplace after being a trailing spouse. Choosing an educational curriculum for her son that might endure each move.

On a satisfaction spectrum of 0-10, where 0 is highly unsatisfied and 10 highly satisfied, feeling 0 for the first 8 months of the recent move.

Finances have been a big part of each move. The need to move for her husband's employment. Shouldering the full relocation cost of doing so, unlike some industries where it is covered by the employer. And also the 'hidden' costs of relocation, such as high health insurance, rental deposits (in some countries a year upfront), interim furniture and large tuition deposits to secure a place. Not being able to afford support such as childcare and domestic help, and not having friends and family to offer it. Not being able to buy a home. Or travel to see family spread across the globe and care for them into their old age. Earning under her potential due to starting again and again.

Primarily, finances affect Liya's ability to protect and care for those she loves most. She fears she or her parents may have to be uprooted again.

And dreams of a smaller world without passports or borders.

Abundance

Abundance is about so much more than financial wealth.

It's about having a rich life. Feeling abundant. Feeling blessed.

One way to feel abundant is to practice gratitude, which is mentioned throughout this book. Practising gratitude fills us up on a deeper level –

and finances become less important. Spending on unnecessary items even less so.

And what's more, practicing gratitude also helps you be more present, focussed, self-loving, confident and energetic. The sort of person that adds value to the world. And in doing so perhaps commanding a higher income down the track too.

Blair's Experience

Blair is wife to a church pastor and mum to four home-schooled kids.

Living 10 years of her childhood in Papua New Guinea, returning home to America, then accepting a placement with her husband on an outer island of Tonga, Blair has had a varied life. She describes her roles as *wife, mom, school teacher, maid, nurse and secretary*. Because you wear more than one hat as a relocating parent.

If it were for financial reasons, Blair and her family would not have chosen this path.

But how's this answer to 'what have you gained by relocating?'

1) The knowledge of a different culture

2) Priceless experiences for the whole family

That's abundance!

Your Finances Action Plan

How would you describe your relationship with money?

Might this relocation change your financial situation?

If so, how will your financial goals change?

Are there others involved in earning and spending decisions? Are you on the same page?

What do you say to yourself when you wish to buy something?

Is there a more positive way to say that same thing? For example, 'I can't afford that' becomes 'I can afford the things I really want'.

In what areas of your life do you spend money in exchange for full satisfaction?

In what areas of your life do you spend money without receiving satisfaction?

What might that spending represent?

In what areas of your life do you receive money by means that give you satisfaction?

In what areas of your life do you receive money by means that are unsatisfying?

What three things could you do within the next month to improve your financial satisfaction?

What three things could you do within the next year to improve your financial satisfaction?

What three things could you do within the next five years to improve your financial satisfaction?

What does true wealth mean to you?

What does financial strength mean to you?

Chapter 10 - Time

'If you're always racing to the next moment, what happens to the one you're in?'

Unknown

Opportunity to do something new

Could this relocation be the reset button? The opportunity to do something new? To reprioritise how your days and weeks are spent? To emerge from your cocoon a butterfly?

There are so many quotes about time.

> *Yesterday's the past, tomorrow's the future, but today is a gift. That's why it's called the present.*

Bil Keane

> *Try to imagine a life without timekeeping. You probably can't. You know the month, the year, the day of the week. There is a clock on your wall or the dashboard of your car. You have a schedule, a cal-endar, a time for dinner or a movie. Yet all around you, timekeeping is ignored. Birds are not late. A dog does not check its watch. Deer do not fret over passing birthdays. Man alone measures time. Man*

alone chimes the hour. And, because of this, man alone suffers a paralyzing fear that no other creature endures. A fear of time running out.

There is a reason God limits our days.

Why?

To make each one precious.

Mitch Albom, The Time Keeper

You could say most of us are preoccupied with time. *Not enough time. Time running out. Rushed for time. Just a matter of time. Being on time.*

We're using being busy as a badge of honour. However busy-ness is a different thing to being productive.

What if I told you you'd enjoy your time more if you focussed less on it? If you practised presence, mindfulness? If you enjoyed the moment you were in?

Perhaps you already do. Awesome! And if you don't, here are some things that may help.

- **Pause.** Whenever you catch yourself rushing to the next task, take a deep breath. Is it *really* that important?

- **Breathe.** Introduce breathing exercises into each day, a few times ideally. A technique I enjoy, via Dr Andrew Weil, is to breathe in through the nose for four counts, hold for seven counts, and breathe out through fluttering lips for eight counts – and repeat three to seven more times. This works for me because I need to concentrate on the counts rather than whatever else is racing through my mind. And it works for my body because it signals to my parasympathetic nervous system that everything is safe in my world.

- **Meditate.** If you are new to meditation, there are lots of free guided meditations you could download off the internet, or buy at a music shop to get you started.

- **Journal.** Allow your thoughts to be freed from your mind onto paper. Perhaps a gratitude journal, or Early Morning Pages, both mentioned in Chapter 1.

- **Slow down with food.** Enjoy the steps involved in sitting down to this meal. Express gratitude. Notice the colours, the aromas, the tastes. Chew each mouthful slowly. Appreciate the quality fuel you are providing your body. Enjoy the company of any others at the table and your own. Put your knife and fork down between each mouthful.

- **'Eat that frog'** a la author Brian Tracy. Get that task you are avoiding done early in your day. Pop it on your calendar as a recurring entry, on mine it is my MIT – my most important task. This one action revolutionised my day when I began. Instead of getting to the end of my workday feeling I hadn't achieved anything useful, despite being busy, my MIT hour of 9-10am meant I could embrace the rest of my day as if it were a bonus.

- **Prioritise tasks** by satisfaction in getting them done. This might be guilt factor, or small to big, or subsequent results. Question any that are not satisfying – do they really need to be done? If yes, do they need to be done by you or could you outsource them?

- **Let go of perfectionism.** Which does not mean not aspiring to do a great job. However, there's often a lot of time between good enough and perfect, and it might only be you who can tell the difference. Join many women before you in becoming a *recovering perfectionist*.

- **One step at a time.** You don't have to do it all at once. What is the next step, the very next step?

- **Do what feels right.** Reassess why something is not getting done – is it because it:
  - is not that important after all
  - needs doing but I'm not the best person to do it, or
  - is a form of self-sabotage and doing it will take me out of my comfort zone, even though I know that is where the magic happens.

- **80/20 rule.** 20% of your time yields 80% of the results. Gain more time by getting rid of some of the tasks that are not yielding results. This is also really good for wardrobe de-cluttering – 20% of your clothes are worn 80% of the time. And eating – if you eat nutrient-dense food 80% of the time, your body will be better able to handle 20% 'sometimes food'.

- **Alternatives.** There is often more than one way to do things. Might a rethink be needed?

- **Distractions.** Shiny things. Say no, even if a good opportunity. Recognise the opportunity cost of saying yes. Might it be at the expense of sleep or exercise or eating well?

- **Plan.** Schedule tasks onto a paper or online calendar. Set goals, break them down into action steps. But allow freedom to enjoy other opportunities that present themselves along the way.

- **Get outside.** Disconnecting from busy-ness and appreciating the beauty of nature is very much underrated. Slow down – and you guessed it, smell the roses. Or watch the clouds drift across the sky, the waves break against the shore, the intricate folds of a plant, the butterfly alighting on a leaf. Time in nature allows you to focus on what is really important.

- **High stress, low stress, no stress.** Our stress hormones are designed to peak when needed for fight or flight, then drop until next needed. Not stay elevated for months and years on end. That's just welcoming adrenal fatigue - and other even scarier health conditions - with open arms. In every week you should have only brief moments of high stress, with longer periods of low stress and even longer periods involving no stress at all.

- **Take time for yourself.** And if that doesn't come naturally, think of the airplane rule – if air masks are needed, fit your own before those around you. You'll be no good to others if you're not taking care of yourself.

Jo's Experience

Jo has lived throughout the UK, Europe, Colombia, India, New Zealand, Australia and Tonga – some locations before having children, others after.

Currently, her roles include mum to two primary-school-age children, wife of a High Commissioner, vice-president of local Red Cross Society, president of her children's school PTA, member of a church and a master's degree student.

Jo is no stranger to being very busy.

When I requested her insights while researching this book, her first response was that of admiration – as I had searched and discovered my purpose soon after arriving. Similarly, she is happiest when using her gifts, fulfilling her purpose.

Jo's advice to anybody relocating – *'give it a year'*. It takes time to establish connections, routines, sense of identity and purpose, on top of feeling the loss of existing friendships. For Jo there were highs and lows throughout her first year in Tonga, even with experience in relocating before, and now she is very happy to be there.

With those challenges come joys – for Jo, meeting a wide and diverse range of new people, watching her children thrive on Pacific island life, becoming an active member of community, enjoying spiritual growth, and having the opportunity to try her hand at new things.

To ensure balance in her life, Jo has needed to let some things go – Facebook is one, blogs another. They were a reminder of what she was missing out on elsewhere. Jo decided to focus on what was positive in Tonga instead – with great success.

And to ensure worries don't chew up valuable time, Jo hands them over to God.

Jo's cornerstones for a balanced life with spiritual growth – family, connection with people, serving the community and faith. As long as I have these, I won't fail. Life is complicated, no matter where I am, how few or how many times I move.

Your Time Action Plan

We all have the same 168 hours in our week.

We also all have different priorities regarding how that time should be spent.

This simple yet insightful exercise allows you to discover if you are spending your valuable time on the things that are most important to you – to your health, your finances, your career, your spirituality, your creativity, your home environment, your physical activity, your meals and snacks, your relationships, your education, your social life - your JOY!

This Time Triangle exercise is also available on the Facebook group Healthy Relocators under files, with a blank template for you to complete.

Grab a piece of plain white paper. Draw a horizontal line a few centimetres from the top of the page. Draw two vertical lines, a few centimetres wide, down the middle of the page. Join the left edge of the horizontal line with the bottom of the left vertical line, at an angle, like a triangle with the point at the bottom of the page. Join the right edge of the horizontal line with the bottom of the right vertical line, at an angle.

Title the left side Actual and the right side Desired.

Note how you spend a typical week on the left side – consider sleep, work, hobbies, exercise, food preparation, errands, family, partner, social, cleaning, meditation, reading, TV, internet, miscellaneous and so on. Where possible, have the items with the largest number of hours at the wide part of the triangle, that is, close to the top.

In the middle column, place an = sign, an up arrow or a down arrow to designate satisfaction or desire for change for each listed item – and on the right side, the time you would rather be spending on each activity (keeping in mind a total of 168 hours).

After completing:

What insights have you gained into your time priorities?

What can you do to make actual time equal desired time for each activity?

In which areas would you like to be more productive or efficient?

Which areas could be delegated or ditched?

Which areas could be grouped for time-savings?

Chapter 11 - Dreams & Fears

'Always put your fears behind you and your dreams in front of you'

Unknown

Feeling fulfilled

There are three ways you can sabotage a fulfilled life.

1. Not following your dream
2. Going the wrong way with enthusiasm
3. Not going in any direction

What are you doing right now?

What is stopping you from following your dream?

This chapter contains a few unblocking techniques.

Karen's Experience

Moving to Australia after 37 years in the UK was bittersweet for Karen.

On the one hand, freedom from family and old friends allowed her to spread her wings and get to know herself more fully. Feeling empowered by the move, she in time established a new business, bought a house so much bigger than the apartment in London, explored new places and enjoyed the beaches.

On the flip side, she missed family terribly, especially seeing her niece and nephew grow up. Until new friends were made, she felt very dependent on her partner, while also initially trapped in a job she didn't like due to employment visa requirements.

Added to the guilt of being a 'bad' daughter and aunt in not being close by, and missing her tribe of long-term female friends, there were wild fluctuations of highs and lows in the first and second year of relocation.

The expense and demands of a long-haul trip to the UK made home too far away.

Four years in, Karen recognises the move spurred her to start looking after herself better. Her relationship with her partner is stronger. She has more confidence and greater quality of life.

Relocating has given Karen the clarity to know what she really wants. She's now creating a lifestyle that allows her to spend two months of the year in the UK with her family, so she can have the best of both worlds.

And in today's connected world, why not?

Wouldn't it be great if …

Once a week, my online calendar pops up with 'Wouldn't it be great if …'.

And on cue, something pops into my head, like 'my email inbox was under 100' or 'I could work outside in the sun today' or 'I had a Virtual Assistant (VA) to do this'.

Then I make it happen. Well, why not? Because that *would* be great.

Fair enough - sometimes my ideas can't happen right away. But invariably they can if I spend some time thinking about the 'how'. Like scheduling a day for an email blitz. Or picking up my laptop and moving it into the sunshine. Or considering which tasks sap me of energy and time, but not that of my talented virtual assistant.

Keen to give it a try?

Sue's Experience

Sue has lived in the UK and three states of Australia.

Getting established and settling up home each time has been challenging, but well worth it for Sue - the freedom, better weather, better lifestyle and improved health consciousness of living in Australia. Family contact is the greatest loss.

Sue's dream would be for her business to be location independent, so she can be free to live and work anywhere. Travel and biz in one.

Give your dream space to reveal itself

Meditate or journal. Read inspirational books and watch inspirational movies such as *The Shift* by Wayne Dyer. Take long walks to allow your inner thoughts to bubble to the surface. Examine feelings of discontent, consider what is driving them. Be true to you, this is your dream, no one else's.

Skye E's Experience

Nine towns in three states of Australia have been 'home' to Skye, she's now loving the weather, resources and parks of Queensland, Australia. Having a partner who works away from home three weeks of every four meant Skye had to make friends and feel understood quickly. A blessing in disguise was delay in finding work – having time for self-improvement allowed her to lose 15kg, boost her vitamin D levels, make new friends, enjoy better health and consider new employment opportunities.

Skye's role model is her mum, as she's passionate and keeps fighting regardless of what life throws at her.

Skye's fear is that she's not enough. Sound like anyone you know? Most people you know?

So she's pushing through that, into a new career, energised by better health.

Imagine what you could do if you tackled your fears head on too?

Your Dreams Action Plan

Here you are going to describe your ideal everyday day. And your ideal 'weekend' day[13].

It's not a plan your ideal holiday exercise. It's a plan your ideal life exercise.

Write down what happens on your ideal weekday. Get creative. Don't limit yourself to reality. Or to the spaces allowed.

Your Ideal Everyday Day

Where do you wake up?

With whom?

At what time?

What is the first thing you think?

What is the first thing you do?

How do you feel?

What are you excited about?

Which clothes do you get into?

What do you have for breakfast?

Kylie Bevan

For lunch?

For dinner?

Where do you work?

How much do you earn?

How many paid hours do you work?

Who do you work with?

How many unpaid hours do you work?

What exercises do you do?

What is spiritual for you?

What is play for you?

What is social for you?

What constitutes 'self-time'?

What is your family time?

What is relaxing?

What contributions are you making to the world?

What time do you go to bed?

What are you thinking as you fall asleep?

What are your dreams?

What are your fears?

Your Ideal 'Weekend' Day

Where do you wake up?

With whom?

At what time?

What is the first thing you think?

What is the first thing you do?

How do you feel?

What are you excited about?

What clothes do you get into?

What do you have for breakfast?

For lunch?

For dinner?

What paid or unpaid work is to be done?

What exercises do you do?

What is spiritual for you?

What is play for you?

What is social for you?

What constitutes 'self-time'?

What is your family time?

What is relaxing?

What contributions are you making to the world?

What time do you go to bed?

What are you thinking as you fall asleep?

What are your dreams?

What are your fears?

Creating Your Future

How close is this to the reality of your current life?

Which items are not too far from reach?

What actions could you take to reach them?

What could you do to work towards achieving others?

How much do you want this?

What would change if your life was like this?

Chapter 12 - The Next Move

'It is only from the valley that the mountain seems high.'

Unknown

Is the grass always greener?

What are the reasons for this next move? Are they solid – or wishful thinking? What are you likely to gain? What may you lose?

These are some of the questions to ask of yourself - and significant others - when considering a move. Perhaps there is no option to do so – if so, are there choices as to where to go and when?

What could you do to ensure you make the best choice? As we've seen in the personal stories throughout this book, having a positive mindset and making the best of what's available is a big part of the puzzle. But it's not everything.

This action plan will help you clarify what you hope to gain, and may lose, from this next move.

Gabrielle's Experience

Australian-born Gabrielle is no stranger to relocation, having moved across Australia and the world five times. Most recently Gabrielle, husband and four children moved to an idyllic, rural location in the north of New Zealand.

It was a dream come true. That never quite felt like a dream.

Instead it was jolly hard work. Sharing a two-bedroom home with her parents for the first month, during a house build. Moving into an incomplete dwelling and washing their dishes in the bathtub. Beautiful land - but more than they knew what to do with. To drive across town was only 10 minutes, after hour-long journeys being the norm in Sydney - but with less options than the city had offered, including lack of variety of people with differing cultural, family and social backgrounds – and difficulties in making real connections with them. It took time to work out where to buy the best, economical foods and products. And also who to watch out for, Gabrielle suggests perhaps like the hierarchy in prison - who can get you what you need, what are the rules and so on.

When renovation costs spilled over and finances dictated a return to work, the commute was suddenly two hours each way – eliminating any time for exercise. This disappointment then led to drinking more alcohol and making less healthy food choices. Stress permeated this happy family. Being so time-poor, she worried about modelling a life filled with work, chores and not much else to her children.

Gabrielle says the gains have been outweighed by the losses in this relocation.

She's certainly gained character - and will go into the next move with her eyes wide open.

Which since beginning to write this book has eventuated – Gabrielle and family will move to the US in 2015.

Louise's Experience

Home for Louise has been Japan, Qatar, the US and four states / territories of Australia.

She's loved the adventure of settling somewhere new, the closeness of husband and kids, meeting new people, finding new business networks, and discovering local places to eat and shop.

She loves where she lives now – and loves where she has lived before now.

Louise is just now beginning to tire of moving. Knowing she has beautiful friends far away. Having to wait for people to start inviting them to things. The initial loneliness. Ensuring the children are coping with everything.

There's another move on the horizon, and Louise knows pre-departure tasks, and first month loneliness are on the cards - but she's also looking forward to enjoying the bonds that form when expat women get together.

Your Next Move Action Plan

Where are you living now?

Where is home?

Where would you like to be moving to?

Why?

Where are you moving to?

Why?

What are you looking forward to there?

Would you like to know more about this location?

If yes, could you interview people who live or have moved there? Google blogs and articles written about it? Read travel books? Go on a holiday there first?

How do you picture yourself in this new location?

Which habits would you like to take with you?

Which habits would you like to leave behind you?

Whether or not your current location is your birth town, what went well here?

What are you grateful for?

*

*

*

*

*

*

*

*

What might you do better next time?

How have you changed?

What did you learn about yourself?

What did you learn about the location?

What would you say to a new arrival?

If you relocated here, what would you like someone to have said to you when you arrived?

How could this next relocation make you a healthier person? A happier you?

So, What's Next?

Self-motivated?

Fired up to make a few changes, to tweak your lifestyle and infect others with your passion for life? Go for it! I can't wait to hear how you're doing and what insights you could offer to others by way of my website!

Share your story by contacting me at my website:
healthwellnessrevolution.com/contact-us,
at the end of a blog post: healthwellnessrevolution.com/blog,
on my Health & Wellness Revolution Facebook page:
www.facebook.com/KylieBevanHealthWellnessRevolution,
or the Healthy Relocators Facebook group page.

Like a little more support?

A small-group program, or one-on-one coaching, available worldwide via Skype, Zoom, Google Hangout, or phone?
Visit healthwellnessrevolution.com/health-coaching-programs/ for more details or to contact me for an introductory session.

Bonus resources

Seeking free resources such as recipes, articles and product information? Check out healthwellnessrevolution.com/free-resources/.

Subscribe to receive even more.

Like to become a health coach too?

Is becoming a health coach your own calling too? I have just the course for you, the Institute of Integrative Nutrition. Questions welcome, ask me and/or the institute, to see if it's a good fit for you. Let them know of my recommendation to receive referral bonuses.

For the men

Have a male in your life who could benefit from a book like this one? Stay tuned. The partner version with specific advice tailored to men, comes out in mid-2015. In the meantime, your XY chromosome friend/partner/family member/spouse will get a lot of great advice from reading this book too.

Success Stories and Testimonials

Julia

It has been a real pleasure working with Kylie. When we met I was feeling exhausted and in need of change. With Kylie's expertise I learnt more about a symptom called adrenal exhaustion and the causes of it and how it was affecting me. I have since changed my diet, have a better understanding of how to manage my stress levels, and feel more energised. Kylie has been instrumental in helping me to achieve this success due to her passion, enthusiasm and insights. I found her to be authentic and sincere. She walks the talk and genuinely wants to help people achieve their own goals.

Before Kylie, I had not been to a coach before and wondered how a coach could help me as I was already good at goal setting. I learnt that it's not just about the goal setting, it's about being accountable and looking at the reasons behind not achieving the goals, if that arises. It also helped me see how limited my thinking had become and how helpful it was to have an 'outside' perspective. I now have a better understanding of how Wellbeing is fundamental to my capacity to enjoy life to the full.

I am incredibly grateful to Kylie for helping me to make the changes that I needed to make in my life and would highly recommend her to anyone seeking to make a difference in their lives.

Kathy

Before beginning health coaching sessions with Kylie I was unsure what it would entail, the cost, time and the commitment. I knew I wanted to be less depressed, lose weight and find motivation to exercise, declutter and set a plan for the year.

By providing nutritional advice and making suggestions I would never have thought of, I am now feeling much more focused and motivated. I particularly like Kylie's friendly and positive approach, and the specific details and links to current research, information and products she provides.

I would recommend her to anyone wanting to improve their health and well-being using realistic choices and information.

Heather

My doctor recommended I look into Kylie's program, as I wanted to reduce my weight, stay committed to achieving my goals, and make exercise an enjoyable habit. After the initial complimentary session, I decided on fortnightly sessions.

I've found Kylie to be a caring and always happy person. She learnt about me, the person, helping me find ways that would work – for me.

Kylie makes you feel good about yourself. I don't want to let her down so it makes me want to stay on track. I know I am capable of achieving my goals, but it is up to me to make it happen.

Kylie is very inspirational in helping you achieve your goals. I would recommend her to anyone I know.

Mary

I'm in my early 50's, had been through a difficult few years with health issues, too much surgery, moved country and feeling downright plump and middle aged and invisible. I also was certain I had psychological issues with food, and had little control over food and sugar cravings.

My first appointment with Kylie was a revelation right from the get go. Kylie suggested (amongst other ideas) maybe I consider going gluten free and see if I felt better. My attitude to that suggestion was 'nah, that's not going to happen'. I left with a revealing book to read Wheat Belly, and that was the moment for me my journey back to wellness started.

Over the following six months, Kylie, with encouragement, kindness, laughter and knowledge, has guided me to a much improved focus on myself, my health, what I eat and a refreshed perspective on life ahead. Her generosity in spirit has been appreciated. I have learnt so much from Kylie.

I feel and look brighter and better than I have in years. I sleep better, have no more hay fever, my anxiety levels have dropped and I feel well armed to make great food choices. Eating well to heal my body has become easy and has happened gently.

Thank you Kylie, your expertise and guidance has truly transformed me and set me on a path of health and wellbeing for life.

References

1. Holmes, T. & Rahe, R. (1967) "Holmes-Rahe Social Readjustment Rating Scale", Journal of Psychosomatic Research

2. www.drwaynedyer.com/

3. juliacameronlive.com/

4. www.louisehay.com/

5. zenhabits.net/

6. leoniedawson.com/

7. www.linkedin.com/in/nataliemontanaro

8. www.marksdailyapple.com/#axzz3CCxwRChb and www.mercola.com/

9. chriskresser.com/how-too-much-omega-6-and-not-enough-omega-3-is-making -us-sick

10. www.youtube.com/watch?v=EOwW9qfW_nU

11. Institute of Integrative Nutrition Health Coach Course Notes: Top 10 reasons to Exercise

12. www.marksdailyapple.com/

13. Exercise concept via Samantha Leith www.samanthaleith.com

Lightning Source UK Ltd.
Milton Keynes UK
UKOW05f0752240916

283706UK00015B/576/P